Everyday Bicycling

Ride a Bike for Transportation (Whatever Your Lifestyle)

Elly Blue

Everyday Bicycling
Ride a bike for transportation
(whatever your lifestyle)

by Elly Blue

First edition first published December 1, 2012
Second edition first published July 20, 2015
ISBN 978-1-62106-905-8

Cover by Meggyn Pomerleau
Fonts by Ian Lynam
Designed and illustrated by Joe Biel
Except illustrations on pages 51, 53, 57 by Ian Lynam
Edited by Joe Biel

Distributed by Legato / Perseus + Turnaround (UK)

Microcosm Publishing
2752 N Williams Ave.
Portland, OR 97227
microcosmpublishing.com

Find this book and more resources at everydaybicycling.com

Also by Elly Blue: *Bikenomics: How Bicycle Cave Save The Economy*

Contents

Foreword to the Second Edition

It's been three years since I began writing what would quickly become the first edition of Everyday Bicycling. I poured everything I knew into it, knowing that much of it might skew out of date very quickly. In the interest of the book aging well, and also following my goal of empowering readers to choose for themselves, I avoided talking about specific bicycle brand names and builds (except in the family chapter where so few options were on the market that naming names made sense).

Revising this book for a second edition, this strategy worked.

A lot has changed in the bike world in the past three years, but the basic mechanics of riding a bike are the same, as are the traffic rules and the best practices for weathering a rainy or hot climate. As I've chronicled in my second book, *Bikenomics*, more people are riding, more communities have developed a thriving bike culture (and have planners and politicians racing to keep up with it), more companies have jumped in to sell transportation-oriented bikes, gear, and clothes. Things are changing: online mapping, physically separated bike lanes, and bike share systems have become more popular faster than I predicted. But your needs as a human who wants to get around on two wheels have still changed. That's what this book is actually about, and it's been a relief to see how well it's held up.

At the same time, change is frustratingly slow. For every family that's joyously starting to pedal around, there's another stuck in traffic on a recently widened expressway on the outskirts of town. It's up to us to make the changes we can, in our own lives and in our communities, and that's what makes the final chapter of this book vital now more than ever. No matter how excited the elected officials, city planners, and advocacy leaders are about bikes where you live, it's up to people like us to lead the way—proving by our pedal strokes that cycling matters, that it is wanted and needed, and that real solutions matter more than symbolic gestures.

My goal with this book is to provide a starting point for your bike explorations. The world is changing fast, and the goal of this book is to empower you to find your own way through it.

The dream I wrote about in the conclusion—that this book will become obsolete—hasn't come true yet. But one thing that does seem to be changing in many places: more and more people are getting on bikes despite what has until now been a fairly narrow cultural definition of the idea of what and who a "cyclist" is. We are learning that we can use bicycles to change our lives, our communities, and the world no matter who we are.

—Elly Blue, Portland, Oregon, February 2015

Foreword

I started riding a bike at age twenty. I didn't have a car and wanted a way to get to work that was faster than taking the bus or walking. Rummaging through my parents' garage one day I found the barely-used purple three-speed bicycle that had been too large for me as a child, dusted it off, and started to ride.

Bicycling was a revelation. I felt free when I rode. I could do more and see more in a day than ever before. But it was also a learning process. At first, I rode everywhere on the sidewalk. I had weekly wardrobe malfunctions until I learned to roll up my right pants leg and ditched my pencil skirts and tight jackets. I sailed through red lights without a thought and had some close calls. My purse straps dangled through the bottom of my front basket and got caught in my spokes. Riding without fenders in the winter, I went everywhere with a stripe of mud up the back of my coat.

I only learned to ride a bike confidently and safely several years later, after I moved to Portland, Oregon. I made friends with other people who rode bikes all the time and who loved to talk over every minute detail of routes and gear and politics. I loved it. From them, I learned to ride in the street in a straight line, to be cautious at intersections, and how and when to signal and yield and merge. I bought lights and fenders and tools and a u-lock and started wearing a helmet. I traded in my heavy old three-speed cruiser for a mountain bike with racks and panniers and found I could carry anything I needed. My proudest moment came when a friend gave me a television and I brought it home on my bike. I stopped asking friends with cars for rides and started riding longer distances just for fun.

Now, fifteen years after I began, riding a bicycle is second nature. It can be difficult to remember that I didn't always know the things that now seem like common sense, like making sure my bungie cords stay out of my wheels and never passing another cyclist on the right. Seeing the huge growth of new riders in Portland and the rest of the country in recent years has brought back those early memories and inspired me to write this book.

Bicycling is fun, safe, and easier and faster than any other mode of transportation.[1] It saves me money, makes me healthy, and above all it brings me joy every day. I learned everything that makes all this possible from the other people riding bikes around me, and am still learning. I want to pass along some of this knowledge to you.

This book is a resource for people who are new to bicycle transportation as well as for those who are looking to make their everyday bicycling experience more awesome. It contains everything that I wish someone had been able to tell me in my first five years of getting around on a bike.

My hope is that this book will inspire you with the confidence and curiosity to continue asking questions and trying new things as you pursue the pleasure of exploring your world by bicycle.

Enjoy the ride!

—Elly Blue, Portland, Oregon, July 2012

---

1 Check out my new book, *Bikenomics: How Bicycling Can Save The Economy,* for more on this.

Introduction

Bicycling for transportation has become hugely popular in recent years. Many thousands of people are taking up cycling, each of them with a unique set of reasons. People ride for fitness, for fashion, to save money, to save time, for environmental reasons, out of political motivations (on both sides of the aisle), for religious purposes, to spend time with friends and family, to remember what it felt like to be young, or simply for the joy of it.

If you've made the decision to start riding, or have an inkling that you might want to, you've come to the right place. This book is intended to help you integrate bicycling into your daily life in a way that works for you, no matter what your reasons for riding are.

I often hear people say, in a self-deprecating tone, "I'm not a real cyclist," "I'm just a fair weather cyclist," or "I only ride on weekends." But any time you get on a bike, that's great. It doesn't matter if you drive or take transit for nine months of the year, or put your bike on the car and drive halfway to work and ride the rest of the way, or keep your riding strictly to your neighborhood. Any time you ride a bike, that's more than enough.

All you need to get started bicycling is a bike and the will to ride it. But bicycling often becomes easier and more fun when you have people to ride with and to talk about all the details with. This book is no replacement for friends, family, and community, but it's a start—a set of ideas and resources to try out, debate, and decide on for yourself.

As you explore the world by bicycle, you will at times encounter people who have strong, and often loud, opinions about every aspect of how you ride. Some of these folks will have been riding longer than you, some will have written books or blogs, some will be industry professionals, and some will just be eager to speak their mind. Listen to them if you like, but don't let their opinions and theories override your own experience, knowledge, and needs.

Most bicycle transportation guides are written for people whose only needs are commuting to and from work. But most of us have much more complicated daily lives and as a result our transportation needs are not nearly so simple. This book is by, for, and about people with busy lives, places to go, and things and people to carry. It is my goal to demonstrate that a bicycle is more than capable of rising to most any challenge.

Let's start by looking at the very basic things you need to know about operating a bicycle on the road. Then we'll help you integrate these bicycling skills into your daily life, choose the right bicycle, and keep it in good working order. My favorite topic follows: how to carry anything by bicycle (yes, anything!). Later on in the book I will turn to the growing community of families who get around by bike to help cover the ins and outs of bicycling with children. And the final chapter is for those who want to improve their communities for cycling, be it through whimsical fun or political advocacy.

Whatever your reasons for, style of, and experiences with riding a bike, don't forget to enjoy yourself!

1

HOW TO RIDE A BIKE

So you've decided to give bicycling a try. Congratulations!

It's easy. It's fun! You just get on the bike and ride.

Right?

Well, sort of.

That's all I knew when I first started riding around town. I wasn't the greatest bike rider, poking along on the sidewalk to the dismay of people trying to walk there. Sometimes I'd get in the street, but I wouldn't always slow down or look first. And I wasn't always very steady on the bicycle. One time, I turned my head towards a distant sound and ended up riding into a wall. On another occasion I was standing at a red light, waiting, and just fell down in a heap with my bike on top of me.

It was only years later, when I joined an email list for detailed discussions about all the minutiae of riding in traffic that I learned how much I didn't know. As I made more friends who also rode everywhere, we talked about what we were doing, what gear we used, what routes we chose, how to be part of traffic.

Once I began to learn, my transition from wobbly novice to confident everyday rider was only a matter of time. I hope this chapter can serve to let you in on some of the basics I wish someone had told me back in 1999.

Learning to Ride

If your last time on a bike was as a kid, getting back in the saddle might be just like riding a bike—or it might not be so easy.

Starting from Scratch

The most difficult part of learning to ride, hands down, will be walking out the door with your bike. Take a deep breath. You can do it!

The best place to learn is a quiet back street or an empty parking lot. Lower your bike seat all the way so that you can put both your feet flat on the ground while you sit on the saddle. Scoot around, lifting your feet off the ground and coasting for longer each time. Have a friend hold on or guide you at first if it helps. But eventually, they'll need to let go. It's counterintuitive, but the faster you go, the easier it will be to balance.

Starting and stopping can be tricky at first. Try to anticipate stops in advance so you can brake slowly, using both hands at once. The rear brake should be your default when you're first learning. The front brake will stop you faster and better, but if you grab it hard by itself you risk locking up your front wheel and flying head-first over your handlebars.

Until you develop an instinct for the bike, your body will want to steer it in whatever direction you are looking. While you're still in the parking lot, practice riding in as straight of a line as possible while looking left and right and glancing back over each shoulder.

Once you're swooping and gliding—and stopping—with some confidence and flair, it's time to start pedaling. Give it a try! Pedal a bit and stop. Pedal a bit more and then stop. Then take a break while you're still riding high on your success, celebrate, and come back the next day.

When you're ready to raise your seat again, you'll have a bit more learning to do. Think of your pedal as a step for climbing up and down to the seat. Think about where you will want your pedals to be when you start again, and plan accordingly. On most bikes you can pedal backwards while you're stopped to get them positioned for a strong start.

In learning to ride a bike, your skill, experience, and fitness aren't important. The type of bike you're riding doesn't matter (though if the bike is too large for you, it will be harder to learn, so err on the small side if possible). The big things you need are patience and confidence. If the person helping you learn is making you feel anxious or self-conscious, ditch them. It's time for you to learn how to fly!

Each new thing will feel a little clumsy the first few times you do it. After that, you'll never think about it again. It might take only ten minutes to learn to ride. It might take an hour. It might take several sessions in the parking lot. You may not get everything right away, but keep going and you'll master the art of bicycling faster than you can believe.

Advanced Road Skills

Riding a bicycle can be amazingly simple, yet there is always more to learn. If you've already mastered the art of staying upright in the saddle, but wish for the skills and confidence to handle every situation in traffic, it's worth continuing your education.

In most cities, you'll find a handful of League Cycling Instructors (LCIs), trained by the League of American Bicyclists to teach adults and youth to ride safely in traffic, through a series of day long classes. Or you might find it worthwhile to become an LCI yourself. If League instruction is not available, the motorcycle skills training course offered by your local DMV can be an invaluable opportunity to learn defensive two-wheeled driving.

For those who prefer to learn on their own, the two classic guides to advanced transportation cycling skills are the extremely detailed and technical treatise *Effective Cycling* by John Forester and the helpfully friendly and philosophical *The Art of Cycling* by Robert Hurst.

Hitting the Road

"My first ride on a bike was scary. I felt exposed and under-protected. Where was my seat belt? I had been conditioned to the comfort and perceived safety of my motorized automobile. I went three blocks, across a busy intersection, then struggled back to my house up a very slight incline. Bicycling is hard work—some of the consistently hardest physical work I have ever engaged in as an adult. This work has had the greatest benefits of anything I have undertaken. It's personal and global. It is about community and self."

—Stacy Bisker, Huntington, West Virginia

No matter what your level of experience is with riding, starting out biking in traffic for the first time will seem new and strange. The good news, though, is how quickly it becomes second nature. You'll learn best as you ride; in the meantime, here are some basic ideas to build on and make your own.

Being Traffic

Here are three maxims for riding a bicycle on the road: Put safety first, for yourself and others. Be courteous second. Third, be legal.

The thing to keep in mind about traffic is that it isn't just cars. When you're on a bicycle, you are not just navigating traffic: You are a part of traffic. So is everyone else in the roadway, whether they're biking, driving, walking, skateboarding, running to catch their bus, getting out of a car, or standing on the corner waiting to cross. Even when someone is not behaving legally and predictably, they are still traffic.

Your job is to pay attention. Notice who has the right of way at each moment. Yield or move forward when it's your turn. Be constantly alert for exceptions, like when someone cuts in front of you and you need to yield out of turn. Sometimes this will mean you'll need to act just like you're driving; sometimes you'll act like a pedestrian; all the time you'll be on a bike.

Not everyone will agree with everything written here. And not everything will apply to every person or every city or every road. Take it all with a grain of salt. Think about it, talk about it, and err on the side of caution when you can. Whatever you do, ride predictably, communicate clearly, and pay close attention to what is going on around you. As long as you remember that everyone else on the road may not be doing these things, you'll be okay.

Choosing a Route

Most people, when they first start riding, choose by instinct to ride on the most direct route to where they're going, the same one they would take while driving or on the bus.

Unfortunately, this is likely to be a fast arterial road that goes straight from your house to your destination. But by all means, if you can ride comfortably on it, go for it. Use this chapter as your guide for how to handle yourself.

Most people don't love these roads, however. They are fast, they are loud, they reek of exhaust, and people in cars don't always expect to see you there and may express that aggressively. If there's a bike lane on this road, it may just be your best bet—but be cautious of those turning cars.

To find other routes, take a look at a map. If your area has a bike map, you may be able to get one for free from the municipal transportation department, an advocacy organization, or a bike shop. Google is increasingly adding bike routes to its online maps, and this can be an excellent tool. If there is no bike-specific map, then find the most detailed street map you can and look for different ways to go.

A friend is even better than a map. If you know someone else who rides, talk with them about which roads they like best and least. There might be a detour that takes you through quiet, residential streets, trading an extra ten minutes of travel time for your sanity. Better yet, ask them to ride with you, at your pace, showing you the tricks and shortcuts they've internalized.

Once you start trying out every permutation of how to get from point A to point B, you'll soon find your favorite ways, as well as the fastest. You may end up needing to get a little creative. The trickiest parts of the route will doubtless be the crossings of busy streets. Sometimes these will require you to make yet another detour, or to get off your bike and act like a pedestrian, or to ride on the sidewalk for half a block. You probably aren't the only person who has trouble with these difficult connections; which may lead you to chapter six for further inquiry.

Always Ride With Traffic, Not Against It

This advice may go against what you learned as a kid. Conventional wisdom used to be, and often still is, to always walk and bike facing traffic, so you can see what is coming and get out of the way. But that advice, like so many childhood myths, turns out to be not just wrong, but dangerous.

Wrong-way cyclists are more likely to get into a crash than people riding with traffic. Why? In a word: Intersections. And one more word: Driveways. People in cars look left before they turn right, because that's where they expect traffic to be coming from. Do you look at the wrong way before pulling into the road? Probably not, as you wouldn't expect that anyone would be coming from the wrong direction, facing traffic. Bu many close calls and tragedies have been the result.

If you live in a city with a lot of one-way streets, it's tempting to ride the wrong way down them as a shortcut. You'll see many people doing this. Often this is because going three extra blocks to always be riding the right way can seem and in fact be just as dangerous, especially when the streets in question are fast and clogged with cars. The real solution to most urban wrong-way riding is to convert one-way streets back to going two ways or to install a counter-flow bike lane.

But in the meantime, I don't advise wrong-way riding for any reason. Nobody expects to see you coming, and police love to write tickets for this.

Neighborhood Streets

Residential streets are often the best places to ride. Car traffic is relatively slow, there's more room to share than on a separated path, you have yards and houses to look at, and people and cats to say hello to.

Even on neighborhood streets, it's a good idea to take the lane rather than hugging the right side of the road. Ride in a relatively straight line, without weaving in and out of the spaces between parked cars. Keep a nice, car-door length buffer between yourself and those parking spaces. Keep your eyes open for people doing neighborhoody things like backing out of a driveway or running in or into the street. And be extra cautious at intersections; many drivers take a casual approach to stop signs on quieter streets. You need to be at least as alert for cross-traffic at intersections where you have the right of way as at ones where you don't.

Bike Lanes

Bike lanes, while they are a beautiful thing, don't guarantee your safety, and aren't always well-designed. Often, the bike lane puts you in the direct path of opening car doors and turning cars and trucks. And in cities, bike lanes are frequently occupied by wrong-way cyclists, pedestrians stepping out between parked cars, taxis swooping in for a fare, unloading delivery vehicles, and other hazards.

On many busy streets, having a bike lane is much better than having no bike lane at all—it reminds drivers that you have the right to be on the road and carves out a small space for you to occupy. But use them with as much caution as you would take anywhere else. Whenever you are in a bike lane, stay alert and be prepared to stop or merge at a moment's notice.

Busy Streets

When you're riding on a street without a bike lane, or if the bike lane is full of gravel or glass, where do you belong in the traffic lane?

Right down the middle of it.

This is daunting, but important.

Many new riders will instinctively hug the edge of the road, no matter how narrow it is. When there's an intersection or a space between parked cars, it's tempting to weave to the right to buy a momentary sense of breathing room before plunging back into the fray.

In fact, the safest place to ride in a narrow traffic lane is nearly always far enough to the left to put you, if there are parked cars, at least four feet away from them—safely out of the danger of getting knocked off your bike when someone suddenly flings open their car door in your path.

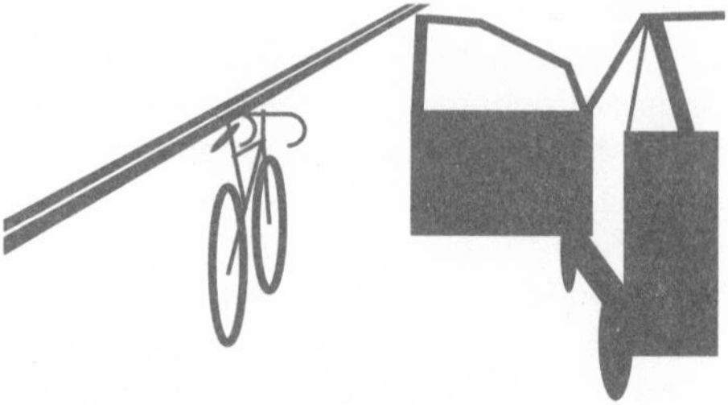

It's a good idea to ride towards the center of the lane even if there are no parked cars. There is a psychological reason for this. When you ride further to the left, your position signals to people driving behind you that it is not safe to pass you in the same lane; they are more likely to fully merge, giving you enough space, or else wait until it's safe to pass. Riding all the way to the right, on the other hand, tempts the person behind you to squeeze past, dangerously close.

On the other hand, when there are people behind you who want to pass and you actually do have space to move over—for instance, an entire block with no parked cars—go for it, it's only polite. Treat this as you would any other lane merge. Check over your shoulder, signal that you'll be moving right, and then move right. Be sure to give yourself enough space to merge back left into the travel lane when your window ends, and do it properly, with a look and a signal.

People may need to wait a minute to pass you, it's true, and some people will get impatient. It's okay. They can pass in the next lane when they have an opening, or when it's safe for you to pull to the right. If the person behind you is not slowing down, or if an impatient line of cars is building up, you can always pull over and let them by. And while I don't recommend weaving between lanes, sometimes riding with a little bit of a wiggle, or frequent glances over your shoulder, can signal to the drivers behind you that they need to give you some extra room when they do pass you.

Taking the lane applies on busy and quiet streets alike. Practice on the quiet ones first, the ones where you are probably going the speed of car traffic anyway. It might feel strange at first, but you'll find that you feel more confident and that people in cars give you more breathing room and act more predictably as well.

If you have a wide shoulder available, then by all means use it. And if there is a lot of aggressive traffic with speeds greater than 25 or 30 mph, it's probably better to find another route. Otherwise, take that lane.

Sidewalks

In some places it is illegal to ride on the sidewalk. In others, it is the only reasonable place. But you're almost always better off in the street. Your chances of being hit on the sidewalk by someone turning in or out of a driveway are higher than if you are in the street. And you also pose a danger to people walking or stepping out of doorways.

If you must ride on the sidewalk, then behave as much like a pedestrian as possible. Ride at the speed of a walk or a slow jog; be alert and prepared to stop at any time. Be most careful at intersections. Stop and look both ways before crossing. Always, always, always yield to people walking; slow down to pass them at a walk, or stop to let them pass you.

Sharing the Path

Off-road paths, rail trails, multi-use paths, linear parks—whatever you call them, they're paved trails, usually along waterfronts or disused rail lines. Originally intended for recreation, they're coming to serve as important bicycle transportation links. On any given day, you'll find people bicycling, walking, jogging, rollerblading, and pushing strollers, often with kids and dogs. Unfortunately, this mix is not always compatible on an eight or twelve foot wide path.

When many people first start to ride a bike, they feel most comfortable on these paths, away from car traffic. They can be quite safe, especially if they are relatively empty of other traffic; but when paths like these are crowded, they are the site of a relatively high number of crashes.

Paths can be absolutely lovely places to ride so long as you treat them with appropriate caution. If nobody's in sight and there are no intersections, go as fast as you want. When you need to pass someone, slow down—to their speed if necessary, and stopping if necessary. Give them ample space as you pass and an audible warning well before.

Just like on the road, you cannot have any expectation of how your fellow path users will behave in any given situation. Assume they are just as likely to swerve or step out in front of you as to move over to let you pass. Likewise, be alert to the possibility of someone passing you, and try not to weave and swerve, or ride side-by-side on a crowded path.

Intersections

Intersections are where most crashes happen. When you're bicycling, it's important to be hyper-aware and to remember that people turning—left or right—probably will not see you, especially if you are all the way to the right, or if it's pouring down rain. It's also important not to rely on people's turn signals or lack thereof. Eye contact, on the other hand, is an excellent tool. Here's a primer on how to handle yourself at intersections.

Turning

Signal your turns!

Signaling is traditionally done with the left arm. Hold it out straight to signal a left turn, with your elbow bent up at 90 degrees to signal a right turn, and down at 90 degrees to show your intention to stop or slow down.

You can also signal a right turn by holding your right arm out straight. This method is subject to debate. Proponents point out that it makes more sense to drivers, many of whom have forgotten their long-ago driver's ed classes and interpret the traditional right turn signal as a wave (or another type of gesture). Opponents point out that you're better off having a hand by your right brake than by your left for emergency maneuvers. I tend to alternate. Whichever you choose, always signal your turns!

Turning right is usually pretty straightforward. Signal, stop if it's called for, check over your right shoulder for crossing pedestrians or cyclists sneaking up behind you on the right, and turn.

Left turns off of busy roads, on the other hand, can pose a sticky situation, since you're most likely to be over to the right. Sometimes you're even required to be on the right. So how do you turn left? When you're taking the lane, you have a couple of options. You can turn just as though you were in a car, signaling left, looking over your shoulder, and merging left in the blocks before your turn, then signaling again, looking again, and making the turn.

If you don't feel comfortable merging—for instance if there's a lot of fast traffic—you can also avail yourself of the practice known as the "Copenhagen left." Stay to the right as you go through the intersection, being wary as always of turning cars coming from behind or ahead of you. Stop at the opposite corner. Make sure you're out of the path of whoever is behind you and then turn your bike 90 degrees to the left so you are facing the direction you want to go. When that light turns green, voila, you're ready to continue ahead.

The Art of Yielding

Yielding is an art form. Who has the right of way? Who goes first?

According to the letter of the law, you should yield the same exact way on a bike as you would in a car. There are exceptions in some states, but for the most part this holds true.

If you have a stop sign, yield. If you have a red light, yield. When in doubt, yield to whoever is on your right. Yield to anyone who is in front of you. Yield to the bus. Always, always, always yield to pedestrians, schoolbuses, and emergency vehicles.

At a four way stop or an intersection without stop signs, the person who gets there first gets to go first. If two people arrive at the same time, the person to the right goes first. If someone is waiting to walk across the street, smile and wave them across.

Be confident in asserting your right of way. But remember that sometimes it's best to yield even when you don't technically have to. If someone's clearly in a hurry, or you're concerned they might not see you, let them go first. Give some extra leeway to anyone who might be angry, confused, or impaired. In all cases, do what's safest and most polite or humane before considering the finer points of the law.

In a car, the culture is all about racing up and claiming your right of way. On a bicycle, it's all too tempting to behave the same way. But you have more to lose on a bike—and more to gain. On a bike, you have the opportunity to yield your right of way with generosity rather than aggression. You can better

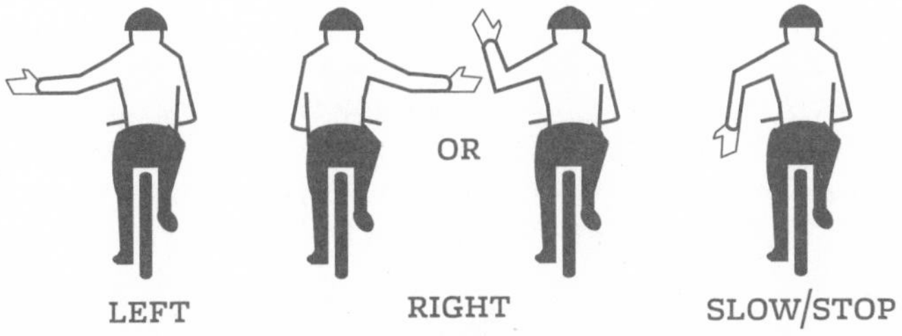

see and hear what's going on around you and correct your course as situations change.

To Stop or Not to Stop

Ah yes. Stopping. In any conversation about bicycling, no subject except helmets is guaranteed to raise more heated opinions. Some say absolute compliance with the law is the only option. Others retort that there's a double standard and that most people don't come to a complete stop while driving. Yet others argue that bicycling is different enough from driving that it doesn't make sense to have the same laws and expectations. Some cities have discovered that when they create safe and clear bicycle infrastructure, cyclists' compliance with red lights and stop signs almost doubles.

When it comes to actual situations on the road, these arguments quickly break down. A strict legalist may roll, slowly and cautiously, through a stop sign. An avowed rebel might wait for a light to turn green even when no other soul is in sight.

Here's a guide on to how to handle the situation on the ground.

Red Lights

Red lights provide clear guidance for everyone on the road. When the light is green, go. When it is red or yellow, stop.

Easy, right? But there's a catch. In many places, red lights are programmed to only turn green when a car shows up. So what happens when you're waiting and waiting....but there's no car?

This was the dilemma that led the state of Idaho, in 1981, to pass legislation allowing people on bicycles to go forward if the way was clear after stopping at a red light. The law was deemed preferable to the expense of retrofitting every major intersection in the state to detect bicycles.

If your local lights can be triggered by a bicycle, then learn the trick of doing this. Usually there is a metal circle or diamond on the ground. If you position one of your wheels to touch part of it, the metal of your spokes and rims should trigger the light to change. If they aren't set up this way, then you have a dilemma. One option is to stop, look, and then go forward, Idaho style, as soon as it's safe, treating the light as though it were a stop sign. In some places, the law allows this. In others it doesn't, in which case you may be legally better off dismounting your bike to cross like a pedestrian.

Stop Signs

Stop signs pose their own set of questions. The other famous component of the Idaho stop law is a clause that allows people on bicycles to treat stop signs as though they are yield signs.

Yielding does not mean blowing through an intersection at full speed. It means slowing down to nearly a stop and making sure the coast is clear. If it isn't, stop. If it is, proceed with caution. Think of it as exactly what a runner would do before crossing a street.

The Idaho stop, though not legally sanctioned in any of the other 49 states, is a nearly universal practice among bicycle riders. When done properly, it can be both safe and polite. But that said, the law often has the last word. Wherever there is police enforcement around stop signs, fines are often very high. If you do not come to a complete stop at a stop sign and then are involved in a crash, any resulting court cases or insurance decisions will not likely go well for you. For many reasons including these, I recommend riding safely and yielding when appropriate at all times.

Other Situations

Road Rage

It will happen. Someone will swerve too close or honk at you or shout at you to get off the road or worse. You'll experience an adrenaline rush, and some combination of fear and anger.

It's easy to rage back. But tempting and cathartic as it may be to return fire with a middle finger or a few choice insults, it's far better not to escalate an argument with someone of unknown temper who is driving a two-ton vehicle. Stop where you are. Walk for a few blocks if you need to. Take deep breaths.

Seize the opportunity to practice memorizing license plate numbers. This can simply be a helpful mental distraction, a way to channel your reaction into something that feels productive. It can be practical as well. If the person was drunk or texting, if they hit you or threw something at you, don't hesitate to call 911. The plate number, the color and type of car, and what the driver looked like will all be of interest to the operator. You have the right to ride down the street without being threatened, assaulted, or harassed.

The Zen of Bicycling

You can notice a lot from the seat of the bike; you see the world from new angles. But at the same time, it's all too easy to get distracted by your thoughts and feelings from the immediate reality of the sights and sounds and smells around you. Bicycling is an opportunity to practice existing in the moment- noticing your breath, your body, your bicycle, and everything around you. You'll enjoy yourself, ride more safely, and be less prone to road rage.

What to Do if You Are in a Crash

If you are involved in a crash, or witness one, call 911 immediately. Get the car's license plate number and the driver's insurance information, if possible. Make sure you get contact information for any witnesses. Call the police and insist they make a report. If you might be injured, get it looked at even if you don't feel hurt in the adrenaline spike of the moment. Write down every detail you can recall before you sleep.

If the other person has insurance, it should cover your medical and bike repair or replacement costs. If you have car insurance, it should also cover you while you're on your bicycle. If neither you nor the other person has car insurance, your own health insurance, if you have it, may cover your bills, and your homeowner's or renter's insurance may cover your bike. Begin the saga of dealing with insurance right away.

If your bike is damaged, you'll need to have it evaluated by a bike shop in order for insurance to cover repair or replacement. Different bike shops will give wildly different assessments, so it's worth going to two or three.

Bicycle crashes occupy a grey area in many bureaucratic procedures. Your situation may not be a perfect fit with the paperwork someone has in front of them, and this can tempt people to cut corners or skip over your case. It's unfortunate, but in many places police, media, insurance adjustors, and juries will empathize with the motorist and assume that the person riding the bicycle was at fault, no matter what actually happened. Insist on being treated fairly, double check every detail, and when in doubt get a lawyer—preferably one who rides a bike themselves.

Sharing the Road with Bicycles

Bicycles are quickly gaining popularity in many places, which means that the patterns and norms of the road are shifting. Below is a brief guide for safely and politely sharing space

When You're Walking

• Stop, look, and listen. You can't hear a car coming... but there might still be a bike coming.

• If you hear a bell behind you, hold a straight line or step right. Not all cyclists know how to pass safely, unfortunately, so glancing over your shoulder and making eye contact if possible is a good idea.

• Refrain from walking, running, or standing in the bike lane on a busy road unless you have no other option.

• When being dropped off or picked up in a car, be mindful of the bike lane. Ask the driver not to obstruct it, and look before opening a door or stepping into the lane.

When You're on a Bike

Maybe you're used to being the only cyclist out there, and suddenly you're starting to encounter others. Here are some rules of thumb for getting along:

• Only pass other bike riders on the left. Never the right!

• Your commute isn't a race. If you have to work hard to pass someone, chance are they'll end up catching up and passing you at the next red light.

• Look sharp at lights and stop signs. Many experienced cyclists are comfortable taking stop signs and traffic lights with a grain of salt; it's easy to develop the instinct of listening for cars and proceeding ahead when all sounds clear. This habit is often so ingrained as to be unconscious, but it needs to be updated for a modern era where you are likely to encounter not only relatively silent fellow pedalers, but eerily silent electric cars. Plenty of damage can be done by either.

When You're Driving

Driving is probably the most difficult, dangerous, and stressful thing that most of us do on any given day. As a result, it's contingent on anyone who gets behind the wheel of a car to be extra committed to driving well. When and if you drive, here's how to be a good neighbor to cyclists on the road.

• **Mind the door zone**. Always look behind you before opening your car door to avoid opening it into the path of an oncoming cyclist. An easy way to do this is to get into the habit of opening the door on your left with your right hand.

• **Slow down.** You'll save gas, you'll save stress, you'll be able to see and react better, and in the case that you do happen to hit someone or something, far, far less damage will be done.

• **Observe the first rule of gun safety:** Never point a deadly weapon at anything that you do not intend to destroy. If you can't see where your car is going, or can't be sure that the space in front of it is and is very likely to remain empty for a suitable distance ahead to match your speed, then you need to either slow down or stop the car. This covers scenarios including nighttime darkness, glare from the sun, snowy, rainy, or foggy conditions, or your own exhaustion and response time.

• **Hang up and drive.** Never use a telephone or portable electronic device while driving. Even using a hands-free headset distracts drivers equivalently to being legally drunk.

• **Watch for cyclists whenever you turn right or left.** Bikes are often in a position to the right of vehicles about to turn right. Left turns are also easy times to miss cyclists. A lot of cyclists learned to ride facing traffic, and others may be acting inconsistently for any number of reasons, so it's a good idea to always keep an eye out in both directions when turning.

• **Pass safely.** Pass a cyclist just as though you were passing another car, leaving them with the whole lane. If there is a double yellow line, a blind curve, or oncoming traffic, do not risk your life or the lives of others. Simply wait until it is safe to pass.

Outfitting Yourself for Safety

You can help make your presence and intentions on the road clear by the way you ride; you can make it even more clear by making yourself as visible and audible as possible.

Visibility

You may have seen her, perhaps just at the last minute—the stealth cyclist, riding down an unlit residential street at night, wearing all black, with no lights, perhaps taking a laissez-faire approach to stop signs. Don't be this person! While there are no guarantees when it comes to safety, on or off the bike, it can only help to make yourself more visible.

You don't have to spend a lot of money or adhere to a certain look. The one key to visibility is, as with everything, to do what you feel comfortable with and what works with your lifestyle and budget.

Lights

In the U.S., most bicycles do not come with lights. Yet in most states you are legally required to have lights on your bike at night or in dark weather. Specifics vary widely—it's a good idea to look up your local statute.

Laws aside, you will definitely need a white front light and a rear light.

Beyond that, the type of light you need depends largely on where you ride at night. If you are primarily on well-lit city streets, then your main goal is to be seen from all directions. Conversely, if your commute takes you along unmaintained roads or unlit paths, then you'll want a super bright headlight that will illuminate the road ahead of you.

Prices range from five dollars for little rubber lights that run on watch batteries to hundreds of dollars for what amount to sturdy, built-in spotlights. If your needs and budget tend towards the latter, be aware of oncoming traffic and turn the beam slightly downward so that you don't blind people.

The most common variety of lights are small, battery powered "blinkies" that clip on to mounts that you can attach to your handlebars and seat post. A cheap set of these are good starter lights, though they break easily, their mounts are annoying, and they tend to get turned on in your bag and run out of batteries at the most inconvenient times.

If you leave these lights on your bike, they will eventually be stolen. I generally clip a red blinkie onto my waistband or bag rather than the bike itself so that I don't forget to take it off when I park. The front light usually goes on your handlebars and is easier to remember. Some people like to attach their lights to their helmets with rubber bands or special mounts. Others hedge their bets with two sets of lights with staggered battery life—one set for the bike, one for the helmet.

If you're stranded on a dark night with only one set of working batteries, the front light is your best choice for them. People driving up behind you can still see you in their headlights if you have no rear light, especially if you have a reflector back there. Your greatest danger comes from people turning off of side streets in front of you. Their headlights are pointed away from you, further up the road rather than at you, so you're harder for them to see.

Nowadays you can get around the battery problem by spending a little bit more on small, detachable lights that you charge via a USB port. As long as they don't get lost or stolen, you'll save big in the long run.

Generator Lights

Generator lights mount permanently to your bike, are difficult to steal, and will never be forgotten or run out of batteries. The standard 60 years ago, today they're coming back into style as more people begin to ride for transportation again and want the convenience of just being able to get on the bike and go.

Friction generators are the classics. A little roller rests against your tire or rim, like a brake, and powers your light when your wheel turns. You push a lever to release the roller when it's daylight. As you can guess, this type of light will slow you down a bit, creating marginally more work as you pedal.

Hub generator lights are the more modern solution. They run off the energy produced by moving parts inside your wheel as it turns, not slowing you down one bit. You will need to buy a new wheel for each light, so these are a substantial investment.

Another type of light is powered by magnets that you clip to your spokes. Each time a magnet passes the light it gets a small burst of power, just enough to flash (many cycle computers work the same way). Some models have a battery built in that can hold a charge for a few minutes so that your lights continue to flash while you are stopped at a light. Magnet lights have the disadvantage of being fairly dim and low to the ground, but are excellent in better-lit areas or if you like to run two sets of lights. They are a value at $45 to $60 per set with no need to buy batteries.

To Blink or Not to Blink

Should your bike lights be blinking or solid? Most lights allow you to choose the setting, and the debate between the two options is a perennial one. Those in favor of blinking lights say that they draw more attention to your presence, and that they only use half the battery power of a solidly beaming light. Those in favor of solid lights demur that these are in fact more visible and less distracting to drivers. The winning argument in my mind is the fact that flashing lights can trigger seizures in people with epilepsy. That's not something I would wish on anyone, and it's all the same to me otherwise, so I tend to let my lights beam out unblinkingly.

Get Reflective

I used to scoff at reflectors and reflective gear—until one night when I accepted a ride home in a friend's car. We drove slowly up a road with a heavily trafficked bike lane on the right. The reflective panels on the backs of panniers, jackets, and shoes, nearly invisible by day, glowed like a beacon in our headlights, far outshining the dim firefly flickering of battery-powered clip-on lights.

In some places, a red rear reflector is a legal alternative to a red rear light, and in others it's legally required. It's good to have one even if you ride with a light—it will never run out of batteries or get stolen or wiggle its way off your waistband to break open on the ground.

Many new bikes and most older ones come equipped with reflectors on the seatpost, on the headtube, on the pedals, and in the spokes. If your bike doesn't have these, look for cheap reflectors in the parts bin at your local bike repair co-op, or new ones for sale online or at a bike shop, often in the kids' section.

For better coverage and more creativity, you can buy reflective adhesive tape in various colors. Several intrepid companies sell kits with pre-cut reflective stuff to cover all parts of your bike, helmet, and gear. You can buy little, reflective stickers to adorn your helmet and water bottle that come in shapes ranging from hearts to spaceships.

Keep in mind that reflectors will make you more visible in a car's headlights—but only bright lights pointed at you will enable someone who is walking or bicycling to see you on a dark road. No matter how well lit-up you are, it's best to never assume you'll be seen.

Clothing

Light colored clothing makes a big difference in being visible at night. As you ride more and your wardrobe evolves, you may find yourself choosing the light green sweater over the dark brown one.

If you want the extra visibility, many sporty cycling apparel companies sell jackets so bright yellow they hurt your eyes and show up in headlights like great green flares. There are many other products you can deck yourself out with, from the bright orange safety vest to reflective ankle straps. As urban transportation cycling gains popularity, there are a growing number of lines of clothing that incorporate reflective fabrics in a more fashionable manner.

For daytime visibility, it can help to look a little out of the ordinary. In some places this might simply mean wearing a suit and tie or a skirt and heels to ride. In others, a top hat or clown suit might be what you need to stand out. See chapter two for more on the bicycling wardrobe.

The Humble Bicycle Bell

If you want to be heard by truck drivers, buy an air horn for your handlebars. For other situations, the classic bicycle bell is the ideal tool for letting somebody know that you are coming along the road towards their about-to-open car door, that are about to pass them on the bike path, or simply to say hello.

All bikes used to come with bells. Back in the 1950s, bells were a part of the transportation vernacular. People simply knew: if you hear a bike bell, move to the right. This is a practice worth bringing back. You can buy a bell for your bike at any bike shop for around five dollars and mount it to your handlebars in seconds with a screwdriver. If you want something that will make a nicer sound and last more than a year, you'll end up spending more like ten or fifteen dollars.

If you have no bell, saying "on your left" prior to passing someone can be effective but be prepared for it to be misunderstood by a surprised pedestrian whose instinct is to step left when hearing the word "left."

Mirrors

Mirrors that attach to either your helmet or handlebars can be obtained for under fifteen dollars.

A mirror can help you see what's sneaking up on you—the city bus with the engine in the back that you don't hear until it's breathing down your neck? A fellow bike rider about to recklessly squeeze by you on the right in the bike lane? On city streets, you need to constantly be aware of what's happening 360 degrees around you. A mirror can help with that.

Or it can hurt. Some people find mirrors to be distracting in the city and not as useful as a full-on, head-swiveling glance over the shoulder. Try it out if you like, and see how it goes for you. But if you spend a lot of time sharing fast, narrow roads with cars that primarily come from one direction—directly behind you—a mirror can be a lifesaver once you've perfected that regular, quick little glance.

Helmets

"I began wearing a helmet when I undertook responsibility toward a significant other, not for myself. I have gotten used to it, and it is a very convenient place to hang a mirror." —R.W., Portland

Based on the data available on head injuries, you would be wise to wear a helmet while riding in a car, running or walking along or across any busy road, and while in the bathroom. But only when you ride a bicycle are helmets not only socially acceptable but considered mandatory. I wear one almost every time I ride and have been particularly glad of it twice. I recommend that you wear a helmet as well, and that you make sure that it fits over your forehead and that the straps are adjusted properly to keep it in place.

That said, helmets are hardly the last word in bicycle safety. Helmets provide limited protection in specific circumstances. They protect you the most in the sort of crashes that typically happen riding at slower speeds and on streets without many cars. Fast car traffic is the greatest threat to your safety as a bicyclist, and helmets, unfortunately, have less protection to offer in the types of crashes that occur in these situations.

Moreover, bicycle helmets have no ability to prevent crashes or create a safer transportation system. And in places where helmet use is legally required, fewer people tend to ride bikes—which has the effect of making cycling less common and therefore more dangerous.

A Final Note on Safety

This chapter should give you an idea of how to ride confidently, predictably, and defensively. These practices, plus some alertness and caution, should keep you upright and in one piece as you go about your day. Helmets can protect you from certain kinds of crashes, and audible and visual signals can help you communicate your presence and intentions to others.

That said, the one single thing that's been proven to significantly improve bicycle safety is the presence of more people riding bikes on the road. That's it. It's no cure-all, but the more people out there on bikes, the more understanding, attention, and respect we tend to get from people driving cars and trucks, and the better able we are to learn good riding and driving skills from each other.

Other research shows that this "safety in numbers" phenomenon is enjoyed not only by people bicycling, but by everyone else on the road. The simple presence of bike lanes on a road has been found to make streets safer for people walking and even driving.

There are no guarantees in life, of course. Using the roads, whether you're driving, bicycling, or walking, is the most dangerous thing most of us do on any given day. But safety is not just a matter of what happens in crashes. Research consistently shows that the risks posed to your health by inactivity, and particularly by prolonged hours sitting in a chair, are far greater than any risks incurred while transporting yourself around by two wheels or two feet. People who lead active daily lives tend to live longer and enjoy greater health and happiness.

So get out there and ride. Do the best you can, and don't forget to have fun.

2

YOUR LIFE, BY BIKE

"It's easier to bike if you have your things organized. If you have your bag and your gloves and your rain cape and your lights all together and you know where they are, you can just grab them and go. If you need to go and you can't find your gloves, you'll be annoyed." —Sara S., Portland, Oregon

When I started riding a bike, I didn't make any wardrobe changes until I had to. At the time I had a professional office job, so I wore skirts, polyester blouses, and jackets. As I biked, my skirts quickly took a beating. The tighter ones split up the seams, requiring emergency safety pin repairs, while the fuller, longer ones got caught and torn in my spokes. As my un-bikefriendly clothes items bit the dust one by one, I migrated towards slacks and flared, knee-length skirts. Cotton blouses replaced sweat-producing (and smelly!) polyester ones. My jackets all were too tight across my shoulders when I reached forward for the handlebars, so I started wearing sweaters instead on days when I biked. As that became more and more frequent those jackets got pushed to the back of my closet and eventually out of my life. These changes happened gradually and almost subconsciously, but eventually all my clothes were far more comfortable, durable, and bikeable than what I'd been wearing before.

Meanwhile, I was making similar adjustments across other parts of my life. Over the course of a few years, without any conscious decision, I started going different places, spending time with different people, changing jobs, doing different types of things for fun, eating differently, and moving across the country to a new city. None of these changes were specifically about bikes, but as I grew older and my priorities shifted, they all added up to meaning I could live the type of life I wanted—and that life included getting around by bicycle.

How Bicycling Changes Your Life

Starting to bike is a bit like getting a major new piece of furniture, a new work schedule, or moving to a new neighborhood. You'll need to rearrange some things and change some habits to make everything functional and harmonious.

Bicycling changes the shape and pace of your life. When you switch from driving or transit or walking to bicycling, it's like you suddenly have a whole different map of your community. Your expectations about time starts to shift, and your ideas about what it's reasonable to do over the course of your day may change.

Some trips will be much faster by bike. You won't be stuck in traffic or on the bus, you can take short cuts, and you won't have to look for parking. The same 15 mph speed that feels painfully slow in a car can be exhilarating on a bike. Bicycling can make your commute time more predictable, and in many cases even faster than driving—particularly when you factor in the vagaries of rush hour traffic and parking.

Other trips will be slower. You might be stuck weaving through back streets with stop signs every block rather than taking the six lane arterial that you're used to driving on. Highways, instead of making your trip across town magically fast, become a barrier that you need to go around or cross.

When you bike, you might start planning your week's errands in advance, leaving more time between obligations, and shifting your daily travel patterns to shorten distances and reduce the number of trips you take. You'll find you spend a few more minutes gathering your things to leave the house—do you have your lights? Is your water bottle full? Enough air in the tires? Is it glove weather yet?

But slowing down doesn't necessarily mean losing time. If you replace a trip to the gym with a half hour commute each way one day a week, you've just saved both time and money. Pedaling your kids to school in a cargo bike rather than driving them adds up to more quality time spent with your family. A ride in the morning can clear your head and make your day's work more efficient and fruitful.

As your map of the city shifts, so will your life. How fast or slow you want your bicycling life to be is a choice that will help determine what kind of bicycle you ride, what you wear, and even where you work, what you buy, and how you socialize.

Some parts of this will be thrilling, others blissful, others deeply frustrating. Sometimes you'll find you want to ride fast, other times slow. Sometimes it's not worth it to bike at all. It's your life and you get to choose how you bike through it.

Work

Recently I met a lawyer who told me that she loves to go on recreational bike rides on the weekends. She wanted to start riding the four miles into work once a week, but was concerned about being able to commute by bike while maintaining a professional appearance.

I suggested that she take a trial run on a weekend. That experience would help her figure out her clothes, her bike set-up, how much time it would take, and what to expect on her route. She wrote back the next week and said she'd jumped in and begun commuting and found it far easier than she had expected—and she was having a blast.

Bicycle commuting doesn't have to be complicated—and if your commute is your major transportation need every day, it can be very simple indeed.

Many guides recommend that commuters wear technical bicycling kits with padded shorts, driving once a week to bring a fresh set of clothes to the office. If your commute is longer than five miles or so each way, or if you are commuting in very hot or rainy weather, this might be your best strategy.

Some workplaces have showers and locker rooms available where bike commuters can clean up and change clothes when they arrive at work. At others, you'll need to manage with a bathroom sink.

For most people, though, all this isn't necessary. Bicycling to work does not have to be an athletic pursuit, and can be done wearing whatever clothes you work in and carrying all your work things in a pannier, along with a rain jacket and a spare set of dry socks just in case. The wardrobe tips later in this chapter should help you to maintain the dress code of your workplace while bicycling.

Parking your bicycle while you are at work may be more of a challenge. If you work in a location with relatively low levels of bike theft, locking your bike to a signpost on the street shouldn't be a problem. Some office buildings and work sites have designated bike parking areas or rooms; in some cities this is required, and it's always worth asking. You also may be able to simply bring your bike into your office, perhaps using the freight elevator.

If your workplace is truly not bicycle friendly, it may be necessary to take creative measures, such as investing in a cheap bicycle that can be parked outside all day, or in a folding bicycle that you can keep tucked under your desk or in the break room. If a bike share system is available and kiosks are conveniently located you may be able to commute by bike without even owning one.

An increasing number of cities offer commuters centrally located "bike stations" that provide secure, indoor bike parking for a membership fee. These are often located next to transit hubs, and some of them provide locker rooms and even showers for members to use and are attached to full-service bike shops.

Shopping and Errands

Commuting to work is hardly the limit of our weekly transportation needs. We must eat, and there are groceries to buy, sometimes in large quantities. There are basic household needs like dish soap, toilet paper, and cat litter. Perhaps you have laundry or dry cleaning to transport. And what about furniture, lumber, plumbing supplies, tools, or a young apple tree? It's possible to carry all of these things and more by bicycle. How to do so is covered thoroughly in the next chapter.

If you are transitioning from driving to bicycling, you may find yourself shopping for groceries and everything else more frequently, buying smaller quantities at a time. This can potentially be more expensive and time consuming than doing big weekly shops at discount stores on the outskirts of town. But when you shop more frequently it also might end up being surprisingly easier and, in the long run, more affordable.

On the other hand, some people, particularly parents of young children, find that when they start bicycling they shop less often, doing as many errands as possible once a week or less, using a bike trailer or cargo bike, or a rental car to haul it all.

As you explore your neighborhood by bike you may end up finding a variety of different options you might not have otherwise noticed. Look for small, family-owned grocery stores, corner markets with a decent selection of fresh vegetables, and specialty stores that sell everything from blank paper to curtain rods to fresh baked bread.

You may find that shopping more frequently and closer to home takes less time than a long weekend outing, and that buying only what you need for the next two days results in less waste. Or you may not—and if you find yourself renting or borrowing a car every week or two to stock up, that's great. It's all about figuring out what works best for you.

Social Life

If the people you spend most of your time with don't ride, you may find yourself as a passenger in a car when you are with them—or they may find themselves joining you on a bicycle.

Sometimes things can get awkward. Some people will incessantly ask, with a pitying tone, if they can give you a ride. Others will assume you don't want to join them in an activity they plan to attend if they can't imagine how you could possibly get there. Some people will lecture you about safety, a panicked note in their voice as they rattle their car keys in one hand. You'll find that many, many people get defensive, assuming that you are judging them for not bicycling also, and explaining and apologizing to you for their own needs and choices.

For all these awkward interactions, though, you'll encounter many others who will cheer you on, and some who will be inspired to join you. Just take it all in stride and keep on living your life the way you choose.

The good news, though, is that bicycling is an excellent way to meet people. Joining a group ride, an advocacy organization, or other cyclists who you meet at work or school or church or on the bike path are ways to make friends with whom it feels normal and comfortable to go out by bicycle to see a movie or take the kids to the park.

Where You Live

You'll soon learn the ins and outs of navigating your way around your daily life. Once you've begun bicycling, it will quickly become clear what works well and what you wish were different. Only a few blocks or one major street crossing can make all the difference in whether or not it is easy and fun to ride from your house to the store.

If you work, shop, visit, or play on one side of a busy street without good crossings, and live on the other, you will likely find yourself thinking about ways to avoid this. Perhaps moving is feasible—just as people will move a few blocks so their kids can go to a better school, others choose to move a short distance away so they can more happily ride everywhere they go.

Moving is often not a near-term option; but you might be able to find a new job, school, or grocery store or laundromat that is more bike accessible (this doesn't always mean it is actually closer). Or your bicycle landscape might just be something you learn to live with. Any situation will become more comfortable over time And you are always empowered to advocate for safer, more comfortable routes (see chapter six).

Where Your Bike Lives

"My bike situation dictates my housing situation." —Austin Horse, Brooklyn, NY

Wherever you live, you'll need to keep your bike(s) somewhere, and often the type of bicycle you ride will depend in part on your facilities at home and work. One advantage of a larger suburban property is you are likely to have extra space—maybe even an entire extra garage—for bike storage. Some imported bicycles, like Dutch bakfietsen, are built to withstand being stored out of doors in all weather.

Many apartment buildings and homeower's associations will not under any circumstances allow you to bring your bicycle inside, and they do not always provide any alternate form of bike parking, secure and dry or otherwise. If you live in a place like this or anywhere with limited space, a folding bike might be your best strategy, since you can fold it up compactly and discreetly and carry it into your home. Using your local bike share system instead of owning your own bike can also be a good strategy, if it's available.

If you can bring your bike indoors, the simplest way to store it is to lean it against a wall. Other bike storage solutions for small spaces range from the brilliant to the bizarre. If your bike has a level top tube, you can make or purchase a sort of shelf or bookcase to hang on a wall, with two notches to hang the bike on horizontally and a handy space up top to drop your keys and whatever is in your pockets. If your bike is light enough to comfortably lift and maneuver, you can hang it by the front wheel from a large, rubber coated hook (a few dollars at the hardware store) drilled into a beam in the ceiling or high on the wall. You can also buy a pre-made, expandable tower that clamps between your floor and ceiling, and can hold two bikes, one above the other.

Wearing Your Regular Clothes

What you wear to bike should be comfortable and appropriate for what you're doing off the bike. If you're biking to the office, wear your office clothes. If you're biking to a class at the gym, wear gym clothes. If you're biking to a party, or to a job interview, or church, or the grocery store, or out on a recreational spin through the countryside, you should be able to hop on your bike while dressed appropriately for each of these activities.

At the same time, not all clothes are great for biking. A polyester blend fabric that keeps you suave and wrinkle-free during an air conditioned bus or car commute may turn into a sweaty, stinking prison on a short summer bike trip. The soles of your favorite walking shoes might be too wide or tall to fit easily on your pedals. The seams on any sort of clothes that you buy at the mall are very much in danger of splitting.

In other cases, you'll likely find neglected items at the back of your closet that become bicycling staples. A pair of wool slacks and a wool sweater can keep you cozy and repel light rain in the fall and winter. Your dress shoes with stiff soles that hurt to walk far in might just be perfect on the pedals. That down vest that always seemed too hot or cold becomes just right on a bike.

Trousers

Wide trouser legs are in perpetual danger of getting caught between your chain and your gears. The classic response to this situation is to roll up your right pants leg before you ride. But there are plenty of other creative options, like switching to pants with tapered legs, or ones that stop at mid-calf. You might prefer to contain the volume of your pants leg with a velcro, neon-colored strap (or a humble rubber band) around your right ankle. Or you could leave your trousers alone and put a chain guard on your bicycle.

Skirts

If a short skirt is voluminous or flared, it's in danger of flying up in the breeze as you ride. Wearing a pair of shorts or leggings under your skirts can solve this problem. A group of women in Scotland developed another technique—they secure a small coin with a rubber band in the center front of a short skirt while they ride, weighing it down just enough to prevent the wind from catching the fabric.

Skirts that are longer risk getting caught in your spokes or brakes, causing a crash. One way to avoid this hazard is to tie the extra fabric on your skirt in a knot or to reduce the flow of fabric by bundling it up and securing it with a large clip of the type that you use in long hair. You can also install a skirt guard over the rear wheel.

Feet

Shoes with a stiff sole will be the kindest to your feet by bike. Sandals and flip flops are often looked at askance, but so long as you aren't racing around and you're careful not to let them flop off into your gears or fall off your feet, you shouldn't have any problems.

High heeled shoes are often maligned for bicycling, but in practice they are actually much easier to bike in than to walk in. The ball of your foot should be centered on your pedal in any event, so the heel doesn't come into play until you need to stop, in which case it makes a nice stilt to keep you from having to climb on and off your saddle.

Head

A cycling cap isn't just a fashion statement, it's functional headwear year-round on and off the bike. The brim keeps sun and rain out of your eyes. A heavier-weight fabric with an earflap will keep you warm in the winter; a lightweight one absorbs sweat and protects your head from the sun in the summer and serves the vital function of keeping your hair from poking straight up through the holes in your helmet.

Layer Up

Depending on the terrain, the weather, and your effort, you'll encounter changing temperatures, both internally and externally, as you ride. Because of this, it's a good idea to dress in layers.

In the summer, you may want to be wearing a sleeveless top for riding, but have a shirt or cardigan to put on as you enter an air-conditioned building and your body cools down. In the winter, it's better to have multiple thin layers that you can shed as you ride rather than a single heavy coat that will turn into a sauna at the first little hill. Arm and leg warmers may look like pointless hipster fashions but are actually quite practical for bicycling, since you can quickly pull them up or push them down as needed, and they provide much-needed breathing room at your joints.

As a rule of thumb, dress less for the weather you see out your window before you set out on your bike and more for maximum flexibility to meet whatever permutations you might encounter throughout your day.

Technical Clothing

There's a lot of fancy technical clothing out there for riding. If you plan to ride more than ten or twenty miles in a day, especially if you like to ride hard and fast, by all means get yourself a full on riding kit: padded shorts, a jersey with pockets in the back, lightweight windbreaker, knee and arm warmers, clip-in shoes and the performance socks. If you like the look and feel of technical bicycle gear, there is no reason not to wear it.

But if you'll be mainly riding for daily transportation at a leisurely pace, this type of gear is rarely necessary. There are exceptions, and many technical items, such as rain gear, have their place in an everyday wardrobe, particularly in inclement weather. But there is no need to invest in an expensive new wardrobe in order to ride a bicycle. Discover what your habits and preferences are first, and choose your purchases wisely.

Padded bike shorts are a popular technical item. If you wear these, you do not need to wear underwear underneath them. Keep in mind that the padding will not necessarily increase your comfort. If your saddle is proving to be painful, your first step should be adjusting the fit of your bike and trying out different types of seats. Try shorts with thinner padding before working your way up to more. (See the section on "crotch health" at the end of this chapter.) If you do wear padded bike shorts, remove them as soon as possible and wash them in between each outing.

Dealing with Dirt and Grease

One of the major clothing pitfalls of bicycling is dirt. There are two main types of bike-related grime. One is dirt from the road, which your tires collect and fling up at you, and the sooty stuff that wears off of your brake pads that begrimes everything they inadvertently touch. The second kind is dirt-infused grease from your chain, which has an amazing ability to get on things that you never even thought came near it.

Road dirt should come off your clothes handily in the wash. Chain grease is another story. If you have a stubborn chain-ring tattoo on your coat (who knows how it got there!), soak the area with a citrus-based solvent, let it seep into the fibers for several hours, and then wash the item as normal.

Chain grease on your clothes can partially be avoided simply by keeping your bike chain clean and well lubed. Dirt from your brakes and tires can likewise be avoided by using fenders and by regularly cleaning your wheel rims with a dry cloth. If it's important to you to keep grease off your hands, keep a pair of rubber gloves with your bike tools and wear them whenever you need to clean or work on your bike.

Your right pants leg is the most susceptible to chain grease. Avoid this by rolling it up to just below your knee while you ride. Or avoid grease entirely (and keep your chain cleaner) by installing a chain guard on your bicycle.

You're most prone to getting dirt and grease on your hands and clothes while lifting your bicycle, for instance up stairs or onto the rack on the bus. Avoid this by learning to lift your bike gracefully, rather than wrestling with it.

One trick is to always stand on the left side of the bicycle while you lift it, away from the drive train. The rest comes with practice.

Riding in All Weather

You can ride a bike through almost any weather. These tips will help. It's essential, however, to trust your inclinations and have a backup plan for extremely inclement weather.

Rain

A light rain, particularly in the summer, can be lovely to bike through.

If it is just drizzling, you may be best off with no raincoat at all. If it is warm out, lightweight synthetic clothing dries quickly, leaving you more comfortable than if you were sweltering in an unseasonable raincoat. If it is cooler out, a thick woven outer layer like a tightly woven coat or a wool sweater is often your best measure; it will shed water and keep you warm even when it is wet.

Real rain, on the other hand, is when technical bike clothing shows its worth. If you own no other piece of technical gear, a bicycle-specific rainjacket is the item to invest in. These are typically made of breathable, waterproof fabric and are equipped with a longer flap in the back, ensuring the small of your back stays dry as you lean over your handlebars. Most have pockets, and many sport zippered ventilation holes in the armpits.

Technical rain pants are another item that many city riders swear by. You can find very cheap, non-breathable ones at military surplus stores, or invest a bit more for breathable fabric and a fascinating array of permutations of zippers and closures. Look for ones that fit comfortably over your regular trousers and that can be taken on and off with relative ease when you are, for instance, standing by the side of the road with a storm approaching quickly.

One of the best and cheapest kinds of outerwear is the rain poncho. One size usually fits all, and attaching thumb loops means the poncho serves as a tent to keep your lower body and feet dry while you ride. If you go this route, you'll really need fenders; rubber boots and/or rain pants are a bonus. The downside of a poncho is quickly discovered in strong winds.

Fenders are essential in wet weather. Water from the sky may get you damp, but the water that your tires throw up from the pavement will cover you with grime. It's possible to buy small, clip-on fenders that will offer some minimal protection, but you'll really be better off with a set of full fenders that wrap partly around your tire and extend nearly to the ground. This is for your own sake as well as the sake of anyone who happens to be riding behind you on a wet day; inadequate fenders will direct a spray of dirty water directly into their face.

Wool socks and tights are especially amazing in the cold and damp, as are any kind of "performance" socks. Neither of these is particularly comfortable when wet, but both are far preferable to cotton in keeping your feet warm.

In wet weather wear shoes with plenty of grip so they don't slip off your pedals. Over your shoes, technical fabric rain booties are nice to keep your feet dry; rubber boots will do as well, though you'll need to prevent water running into them from above.

As for keeping the rain out of your eyes, a visor on your helmet will help marginally; a cycling cap with a brim will help even more. You can also purchase a waterproof helmet cover to keep your whole head somewhat more dry and warm. Some rainy weather riders prefer contact lenses over spattered and fogged glasses.

A note about size: Technical bike gear, including rainwear is rarely made in women's sizes above 14. You'll find a few things out there, but the options are limited. If you have trouble finding rain gear that fits you, a poncho is one option; or you may prefer to swing the opposite direction and opt for a fashionable wool or waxed burlap coat.

Cold

People who ride frequently in colder climates recommend dressing so that you feel cold when you leave the house, in order to achieve the perfect temperature during your commute.

In staying warm, you have two factors to consider. First, if you are riding hard, your body will warm up. But at the same time, when you ride the air will rush by you—especially if it's windy—making it feel much colder, especially on your hands, feet, and face.

Most warm winter clothing focuses on keeping your core warm—a giant down jacket, for instance. But your core is what heats up the fastest when you're on a bike. Get too warm, and you'll find your sweat cooling you down too fast when you stop riding.

Keep in mind that in any kind of cold weather, your main concern should be staying warm rather than staying dry. Sweat can freeze as well as any precipitation, so the trade off between internal and external moisture must be balanced.

So unless you are riding in below-freezing temperatures, ditch the parka and layer up. This might entail a lighter jacket over a couple of sweaters, and long underwear underneath all your clothes. You'll also want more, warmer coverage of your extremities, for instance double socks, gloves, scarves, and hats.

Pay extra attention to the gaps between items of clothing that are exaggerated when cycling: at your neck, between your gloves and sleeves, at your ankles, and your lower back between your waistband the bottom of your shirt.

Military surplus stores are excellent places to get cold weather biking gear along these lines, particularly wool.

Snow and Ice

People who ride in snowy climates often keep separate bicycles that are set up for winter riding. Variations abound. For some kinds of snow, knobby mountain bike tires may help you gain traction. But on ice or hard packed snow, smooth tires are better as they provide more surface area to grip the slippery road. In slippery conditions, lowering your tire pressure to its minimum may also help increase the amount of gripping surface on your tires. Just like for a car, it's possible to purchase (or make) studded tires for your bike. For slushy or sticky snow, you might want to lose the fenders you needed for the rain or wintry mix earlier in the week.

For comprehensive advice about cycling through hard winters, the long-running icebike.org website maintains the best resource that I know of, and is also home to a helpful email discussion list.

Heat

There are two schools of thought about bicycling in very hot weather. One is to wear as little as possible to stay cool; the other is to cover up with lightweight fabric to avoid sunburn. Cotton is more comfortable and breathable, and lightweight wool designed for athletic activity has its devotees. Whatever you wear, light colors will absorb less heat.

Drink a lot of water when you're biking in hot weather. Several cups of water before you leave the house will get you started, and then drink more as you ride. Drenching your hat and shirt in water before a ride in the scorching heat can help your body keep cool for longer.

Sweat is a concern for many people transitioning to a bike commute. One way to reduce the amount you sweat is to give yourself enough time to always ride slowly; give yourself time to coast and feel the breeze! If you are simply a sweaty person, use that extra time to freshen yourself up in the restroom when you arrive. Tying a handkerchief or silk scarf over your hair and under your helmet can help keep it in order, but in general you'll find it easier to skip the heavy makeup and elaborate hair regimens in summer. You can make your sweat smell a little sweeter by drinking a lot of water and avoiding greasy foods.

Also, it's counter-intuitive, but steering clear of heavy air conditioning will help your body acclimate to the heat. It takes about two weeks to really get used to hot weather, and every blast of AC resets the clock. So it sounds strange, but if you must spend any amount of time in a chilly air conditioned place in the summer, wearing a warm sweater while indoors will help you be more comfortable when you leave.

Plan your day to stay cool. Where I live, peak temperatures are reached between 4 and 6pm—right during the evening commute. If you can avoid traveling during the hottest time of day, do so.

Whatever you do, take it slow and easy when it's hot. And when you put on sunscreen, don't forget that exposed stripe on your lower back.

Take Care of Your Body

Bicycling doesn't have to be an athletic endeavor, but it is undeniably a physical activity. When you begin to bike regularly, you may find you simply need to eat more throughout the day to avoid the dreaded blood sugar crash that athletes refer to as "bonking." Making sure some of those extra calories consist of fresh, whole foods will give you more energy and strength for riding. Always having snacks on hand can be a lifesaver.

Stretch and Strengthen

Muscles get tight when you use them. Your body will thank you if you stretch regularly, even if just for thirty seconds or a minute before or after a ride or at the end of your day. Yoga is especially good for staying limber and strong, but the basic stretches you learned in gym class as a kid will serve just as well. Your hamstrings, quads, and hips in particular will thank you for stretching them.

Bicycling gives you strong legs, but it doesn't do much for your upper body strength or your core. Any form of exercise that builds abdominal strength will help you get up those hills. Improving your overall fitness will make bicycling continually easier and more fun, so if it feels good, go for it.

Finally, riding a bike should never hurt. If you're in any kind of pain, something's wrong. You might need to start stretching a particular muscle, tweak the fit of your bike, adjust your saddle, get your cargo off your back, try a new kind of handlebar setup, or even see a doctor. Regardless, don't just push through the pain; research it and consult an expert.

Crotch Health

A few sensational articles have been published over the years claiming that cycling can harm your sexual health. And if you ride for many hundreds of miles each month you are indeed likely to suffer in the crotch department. If you are a more casual rider, however, you need only worry about your fertility and nerves if you actually experience discomfort or numbness.

When you first start riding, or when you switch to a new saddle, the bones in your pelvis will probably be sore for a few days. This is normal; if it is deeply painful, or doesn't fade in a week, adjust your saddle or switch to a different one.

To stay comfortable in the long term, it's important that your bicycle and all its parts be well adjusted for your body. This is not just a matter of your saddle adjustment; even a centimeter's difference in the angle of your handlebars can affect the comfort of your seat. For more on bike fit, see chapter three.

Experiment with different clothes and equipment to make sure you are not over- or under-padding either your bicycle seat or your crotch. Some people can ride effortlessly, wearing anything and on any saddle; others are most comfortable with lots of padding, others with thin padding, others with none at all. Some people find that any clothes with seams in the crotch, particularly jeans, are unbearable to ride in. If you experience lasting numbness or pain, see a doctor and switch to a different type of bike.

Gel can bunch up against the soft tissues, producing painful results. There is a vicious cycle that many riders fall into; their initial saddle is uncomfortable, so they get padded shorts. But they are still uncomfortable, so they get new shorts with thicker padding, and when this doesn't help they also get a gel padded seat and then eventually give up riding entirely or even undergo surgery to attempt to solve the problem. I started down this road myself and fortunately did not get very far before I forgot my padded shorts for a 65 mile ride, which is much longer than I ever typically ride. I completed the ride in leggings and at the end, every part of my body hurt except my crotch. I ditched all my bike shorts and saved myself a good deal of pain and money since.

Also in the crotch department, it's important to be extra attentive to hygiene. This is especially true if you wear synthetic underwear or technical bike shorts, which are ideal bacterial and yeast breeding grounds. If you do go for long rides in bike shorts (or ride any distance in warm weather with any synthetic fabric next to your skin), keeping very clean and using a chamois cream (it's pronounced "shammy") can help prevent painful chafing and saddle sores. After a sweaty ride, products like Bag Balm can relieve chapping.

Menstruation

Many women find that menstruation does not affect their bicycling routine in any way. Some enjoy reduced cramps and premenstrual symptoms as a result of bicycling and generally staying physically active. Other women find that their period brings a low ebb in energy and an increase in physical and mental discomfort such that they are better off taking a break from bicycling—and everything else—for a day or two.

As for dealing with the actual flow, this also varies, and tends to only be a problem for those who have heavy bleeding. Some women avoid using tampons when they bike, finding them uncomfortable and less effective. The tampon string in particular can be chafing; snipping it off helps. A popular alternative is the reusable menstrual cup. Multiple varieties are on the market, made of either rubber or silicone.

Pads pose a different issue. Thicker disposable pads tend to bunch up uncomfortably. The extra-thin variety work better but suffer extra wear and tear in the saddle and will need to be changed more often than is typical. Cloth pads are not usually ideal; they are either too thick or they shift around while you ride. Some varieties are secured with a snap, which is not well placed for comfort on a bicycle seat. Some types of thinner cotton pads with an impermeable backing and with a non-snap closure do exist, but can be difficult to source reliably.

Going Multimodal

When you choose to hop on a bicycle, that doesn't mean that bicycling is the only way you'll ever travel again, ever, or even on a daily basis.

Public Transportation

Public transportation and bicycling can be a winning combination. Transit lines are only convenient if you live near one stop and are going somewhere near another one. Bicycling can help you bridge the gap. If you can bike for several miles, you can skip some connections and avoid the hours-long bus rides to go a relatively short distance that often make transit unfeasible.

In many places, you can bring your bike onto the bus or train, though sometimes this is only allowed during limited hours, or if there is room on board in the designated bicycle spaces.

If bringing your bike on the train or bus is a problem, you have two options, cheap and expensive. The cheap one is getting a beat up but ride-able bike and locking it up out in the elements at your transit stop. The more costly option is to invest in a folding bicycle. These bikes fold down small enough to bring with you on public transportation without too much trouble, and nearly all transit systems allow them. The best quality ones are quite comfortable and fast to ride and some even have racks so that you don't need to wear your things on your back.

Cars

You might curse the existence of cars while you're trying to share a busy road with them. But with so many places built with automobiles in mind, sometimes you just need to use one. When you also have your bike with you, that can pose some interesting logistical issues.

The easiest way to transport most bicycles in a car or taxi is in the trunk. Remove the wheels, rest the frame in the trunk with the gears facing up, and place the wheels in on top of it. If you don't have time or the right tools to get the wheels off, you can still put your bike in most car trunks. Slide the bike in with the back wheel first, gears facing up, and leave the front wheel and handlebars hanging out the back of the trunk, rotated at more or less 90 degrees. Bring the trunk lid down gently onto the frame. If you are going far, fast, or over bumpy streets, use a bungie cord, a rope, or even your shoelaces to secure the trunk lid snugly so it doesn't bounce open and closed while you drive.

If you find you are often driving with your bicycle, it may be worthwhile to invest in a rack made for the purpose. Many a rural or suburban commuter has discovered they can get their bike commute in and save money on inner city parking by driving part of the way, parking in a lot or a residential street, and riding the rest of the way into work. With a rack, you can bring bicycles with you on a road trip and explore a new city or campground without the frustrations of driving.

I recommend bicycle racks that attach to the back of your car rather than the top. It is easier to get the bikes on and off, to lock and unlock them, and you can easily remove the rack when you aren't using it. You'll also avoid the danger of forgetting that your cargo is taller than a bridge clearance or garage door. Affordable, used racks in good condition are easy to find. If you leave your bicycle unattended on either kind of rack, be sure to lock it securely.

Traveling by Bike

Traveling long distances? It can still be done with a bicycle. Bringing a bike on an airplane is cumbersome and expensive, but some airports are beginning to encourage bicycle connections by providing safe, well-signed routes and even tools for disassembling and boxing up your bike. Others will actively discourage you from riding to the airport. Most long distance trains and buses allow bicycles; some require you to box your bike and others don't. Triple-check the rules before you go; often there are different requirements and fees for different lines and stations. If you have a folding bicycle, your long-distance travel connections on any mode will be greatly eased.

Or you can just do all the traveling by bike. Bicycle touring is enjoying a renaissance in North America, with thousands of people each year pedaling across the country, around the world, or just on quick camping trips near their homes.

3

BICYCLE ADOPTION, CARE, & FEEDING

For years, I kept only one bicycle at a time. First it was a series of vintage cruisers, then a mountain bike converted to city use, then a fast, custom road bike, and finally that mountain bike again, converted to a longtail cargo bike.

I have loved both of these bikes more than I can say and ridden each of them many hundreds of miles. But there have also been times when each one filled me with frustration and stress. I've been guilty of what I now realize is a common mistake: Demanding that one single bicycle be and do everything.

The custom road bike was perhaps the most intense example. It was expensive and it was made for me, so my expectations were particularly vast. I loved going fast, but whenever I took it out, I needed to carry a lot of heavy things. The bike was made to fly, not haul, and the heavier the load, the more unbalanced I felt.

It stopped being fun to ride, so I lent it to a friend and got a cargo bike instead. The cargo bike perfectly suited my lifestyle and was all bliss for a while—I could carry anything at all!—but soon enough the frustration was back. When I was riding with others, I couldn't keep up. A quick trip across town took fifteen minutes longer than I felt it should. The joy of being able to carry anything at all under my own power gave way to the irritation of crawling along even when unencumbered.

So I brought home the fast bike, took the racks off, and vowed to never again push a bicycle to be something that it wasn't. Now, when I want to carry anything beyond snacks and my wallet, or if I just feel like sitting upright and tootling along slowly, I ride the cargo bike. When I want the thrill and athleticism of going fast, I put all my errands aside and treat myself to a spin on the road bike.

There are times when one bike is in the shop, and I ride the other for every purpose, and that's liberating in its own way, remembering how far you can push a bicycle. But having two bicycles works well for me—so well that I eventually bought a third bike, a folding bicycle that can travel anywhere by train or car and sturdily and steadily carry me and all my things all around the destination.

Complicated Bikes for a Simple Life

Bicycling can be as simple or as complicated as you want it to be. Much of that depends on your choice of bike.

If you walk into a bike shop and ask for the simplest bicycle they have, it's likely they'll direct you to a row of minimalist stripped-down, fast steeds without gears and brakes, much less a rack or fenders. These bikes are easy on the wallet and fun to ride but can end up complicating your life on a daily, practical level, requiring extra creativity and effort to manage even simple tasks like grocery getting and riding in the rain.

If you want to keep things truly easy and change your daily habits and dress as little as possible, consider going for a more complicated bicycle. A bike with some combination of sturdy step-through frame, built-in lights, fenders, a chain guard, a rack, and flat-resistant tires will not be your fastest or lightest or sleekest choice, but it will simplify your transition to bicycling immensely. It is a shame that most bike shops don't sell ready-made commuters fitted out with all of these items—the simplest bike of all is one that is ready to meet all the challenges of your daily transportation needs without increasing your cognitive load with a bunch of decisions and options.

There's something to be said for complexity, too, though, and you may find, as you ride more, that you enjoy the learning and the trial and error of tinkering with your bicycle and tailoring it to fit your body and lifestyle. This chapter gives you some very basic resources to whet your curiosity and get you started.

Choosing a Bicycle

"Don't try too hard to get the right bike from the start. Tastes change with time, experience and fashion" —*Erik Sandblom, Göteborg, Sweden*

What kind of bike do you need? The short answer is: Any kind. It doesn't matter, so long as you can ride it.

The longer answer is: You need a bike that you like, that fits you, that can be kept in good repair, that is suited to your life and the terrain you'll be bicycling over, and that is fun to ride.

Within those parameters, you'll find multiple options, sometimes too many. Keep in mind that there is no single ideal bicycle. Choosing a bike is a matter of figuring out your needs and then finding a bike that will suit them reasonably well.

If you already have a bicycle, skip ahead to the maintenance section in the second part of this chapter. If you have a search ahead of you, here are some tips for choosing your bike.

You Don't Need to Marry Your Bicycle

Don't assume you need to have the ideal bike before you start riding. Waiting for the perfect bike to come along is a great recipe for never beginning to ride at all. Another pitfall is that when you do find the dream machine that fits all your initial criteria, it is likely to be a hefty investment. If this expensive new bicycle turns out to not be a good fit for your body or your lifestyle, you're bound to feel frustration instead of joy when you ride it.

Avoid this fate by shopping around with the goal of honing in on your needs. If you already have a bike that you aren't thrilled with, think about what could make it more fun to ride and make incremental changes one by one with that end in mind. If you're totally new to riding, one way to get started is to borrow a bike from a friend or family member who is about your height. Even just renting a bike for an afternoon or test riding a different style of bike at your local bike shop every weekend will help you get a sense of what you like—and, just as important, what you don't like.

Then again, if you know you want to ride, there's something to be said for just jumping into the deep end and getting yourself a bike, any bike. Why wait? Bikes have good resale value, and the bike that frustrates you daily is likely someone else's dream ride. If your shiny new ride doesn't work out, you can always sell it and get something else. The real risk is never getting started, or torpedoing your whole bicycling future because in frustration at one ill-fitting steed.

You don't have to marry your bike. If your first bike ends up not being right for you, there is no shame in that. Adjust it until it fits your needs as well as it's going to, and then take what you've learned and move on. For most everyday riders, life is a never-ending quest for the perfect bike set-up, which is often approached but never achieved. There's joy to be found in that, too.

New Bikes

New bikes have advantages and disadvantages. They are in one sense easier to shop for, because they are standardized; you will not be faced with a multitude of individual quirks and component choices. A new, low-end hybrid commuter bike is an easy and affordable entry into the world of cycling, and can be passed along to another new cyclist or resold for a reasonable sum when you are ready to move on.

Low-end new bikes are not to be confused with their cheaper cousins the big box store bikes, which are as a rule not built to withstand regular transportation use. If you are unsure that you want to ride at all, and only want to spend a hundred dollars testing the waters, a big box bike might be a temporary solution. Keep in mind that these bikes do not have any resale value, and are very difficult to maintain due to various key parts being made of plastic. There is a danger that this type of bike will be so rickety right out of the box that it will put you off riding entirely. Proceed with caution, and if you do choose this avenue, plan to replace the bike within six months.

Working with a Bike Shop

"Ask friends and/or the Internet for recommendations for good bike shop. Tell a shop the kind of riding you plan to do and any physical issues." —Lisa F., Portland, Oregon

You can save money by buying a bike online but if you'll be riding regularly, it's worth spending a little extra in order to develop a relationship with your local bike shop. That way, when your new bike hurts your wrists or develops a rattle in the first week, you'll have ready help adjusting it to fit and making sure you are happy. You'll always have a place to go with questions, fit help, and repair needs, and when you're ready to buy another bike you'll have the advantage of a guide to the process who is already familiar with your needs.

If there are multiple bike shops in your area, it's a good idea to shop around. You'll want a place you feel comfortable and where they have the things and services you need in your price range. If you have a good interaction with a particular employee, it's fine to ask for them specifically when you go back.

Bike shops can be intimidating to the uninitiated—but they don't have to be that way. To have a positive experience, there are three rules of thumb:

1. Be prepared. Go in with as clear an idea as possible of what you need, whether this is the exact part number or just "I want a red bike that is fast and reliable." Even if you don't know where to begin with researching your needs, think them through as thoroughly as you can. Your bicycle dreams will evolve along with your knowledge.

2. Ask questions. If the salesperson or mechanic says something you don't understand, ask them to clarify. If you do happen upon someone who isn't willing to answer your questions or who doesn't listen, find another employee to work with or go to a different shop.

3. Test ride, test ride, test ride. Never purchase a bicycle that you have not first taken for a spin and found to be comfortable.

Used Bikes

"If you are concerned you may eventually be dissatisfied with new bike, a used bike will be easier to sell for the purchase price."

—Austin Horse

There are many good reasons to buy a used bike. A well cared-for bike that has already lasted many miles will likely last many miles more. And as with so many manufactured goods, older bikes and parts are better-made than many of their newer counterparts.

Another benefit of a used bike is that vintage bikes are often better-suited for city riding. If three gears are enough for your purposes, then a vintage three-speed with a good-condition, internally-geared hub will need less maintenance and result in fewer surprises and breakdowns.

Used bikes, unless you buy them from a shop that restores them lovingly, may need some initial investment beyond the purchase price. If you purchase a bike that has been sitting, lonely, in someone's garage for several years, you will likely need to replace the rubber bits on it—tires and brakes—as well as the shifting and brake cables. You may also find that other parts of the bike, like the chain and gears, are worn out and need replacing. Test the bottom bracket by holding a pedal in each hand and wiggling them to make sure they are sitting tightly in the frame.

Steel frames are heavier, but will last for decades. Aluminum and carbon are less durable and can't be repaired. Before you pay for the used bike you've chosen, run your eyes over every centimeter of the frame. Look for dents, cracks or signs of strain—if you see anything like this, move on.

You may end up spending as much as two or three hundred dollars extra fixing up a used bike—but this can still be an excellent bargain for a bike that is a joy to ride and will last you for years.

It's also worth noting that you might be able to find yourself a used bike for free or very cheap at a community bike shop. See the Maintenance section of this chapter for more information.

Types of Bicycles

The variety of types of bicycle out there is bewildering. Below are some of the basic types. But don't worry about brands and categories too much; the lines between them can be blurry and are often defined more by industry marketing than by actual features. What matters is that you have a bike that fits you, that works for you, and that you enjoy riding.

City Bikes

Just what is a city bike? There is no single answer. In essence, though, it's a bike suited to everyday urban cycling, as opposed to other specific uses like long, recreational rides in the country or racing on tracks or down mountain trails.

A classic European-style city bike has full fenders, a rear rack, and perhaps a front basket. It might have a chain guard and perhaps it also has a skirt guard: A casing over the rear wheel that keeps your skirt or coattails out of the spokes. A city bike likely offers an upright riding

posture and a step-through frame. It almost certainly sports a bell and may have integrated generator lights.

In North America, bikes adapted for city riding tend to look a little different from this European ideal. They are often road bikes fitted with handlebars that allow a more upright posture, racks, fenders, wide tires for a more stable ride, and perhaps built-in lights. Almost any bicycle can become a city bike; the permutations and possibilities are endless. The shop that sells you one might call it a Dutch bike, a commuter, a cruiser, or a hybrid, depending on what sort of bikes they carry and what they think their customers want.

A Note on Step-Through Bikes

When you think of a bicycle, the image that first comes to mind is likely of a diamond frame road bike, with a straight top tube between the seatpost and the handlebars.

While diamond-shaped frames tend to be thought of as men's or boy's bikes, step-through frames, which lack the straight top tube, have become branded in the U.S. as girls' or women's bikes. They were indeed invented for women in the late 1800s, meant to accommodate riding in long, heavy skirts and petticoats. Clothing norms have changed, but the association of step-through bikes with women and diamond frame bikes with men remains.

There is no reason today for people to choose a frame style based on gender. People who want to ride fast tend to prefer diamond frames, while step-through frames (you might also hear some varieties called loop frames or mixtes) are ideal for people of any gender who carry children or cargo on their rear rack, interfering with their ability to swing their leg over the back of the bike. Step-through riders can also include people with hip injuries and anyone who simply wants the ease and freedom from wardrobe malfunctions of being able to simply step in front of their handlebars and ride.

Dutch Bikes

If you ride short distances, prefer to wear fashionable clothes on your bike, don't have many steep hills to traverse, like to take it slow and smell the roses, and don't want to ever to do any maintenance, then an upright Dutch-style bike with just a few gears may be right for you.

Imported Dutch bicycles are still rare in the U.S. but they are gaining in popularity. They are often but not always step-through frames. They allow you

Be Prepared

Before you go bike shopping, think about the following questions. Maybe take some notes.

- Do you want to ride fast or slow?
- How far will you be riding, and how often?
- Are there a lot of hills where you will be riding?
- What kinds of roads will you be riding on—smooth asphalt, rutted streets, or gravel/dirt roads? Will you spend a lot of time on busy streets?
- What do you want the bike to look like? It's okay to care about style and color!
- Will you be carrying stuff on racks on your bike? Will you use a trailer with it? Will you carry children?
- Will you need to carry your bike up and down stairs?
- Where will you park?
- How much do you want to spend?

Even if you do not yet have answers to all of these questions, considering them will better equip you to begin shopping for a bike that meets your needs.

to have a bolt upright riding posture as though you were sitting on a chair or riding a horse. They tend to be heavy, sturdy, and usually do not come with very many gears, since most of them are still imported from the pancake-flat Netherlands. They also tend to come equipped with components suitable for city riding including built in fenders, lights, chain guard, and a dress or coat guard. They are an expensive option in the U.S. but that may change as cheaper imitators enter the market.

Road Bikes

If you are always on the go, need to hop between commitments all over town, live in a walk-up apartment, aim to replace your gym membership with your daily riding, or want to be able to flip your bike over and fix it on the fly, a light, fast road bike might be for you.

Road bikes are diamond frame bikes, and they typically come with s-curved "drop" handlebars that require you to bend forward to ride. They can be excellent transportation

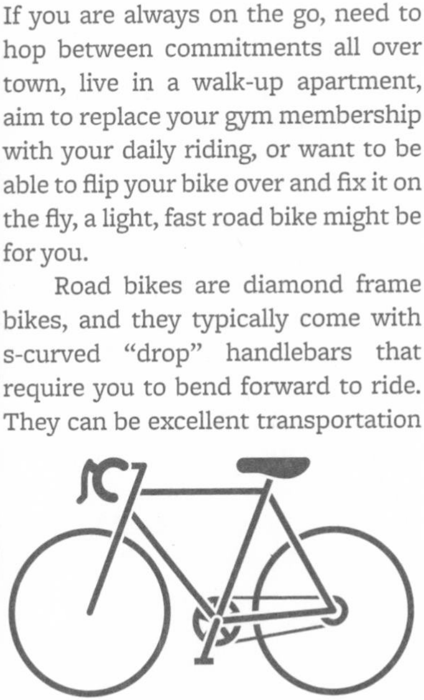

bikes, especially if you prefer speed. When shopping for a road bike, consider that you may want to attach rear fenders and a rear rack. Not all road bikes have the proper attachments that make this process straightforward. Also, many people enjoy the bent-double, aggressive riding posture of a road bike, but it is not practical or comfortable for everyone. If you want a road bike but prefer to sit more upright, consider tilting your handlebars up higher, adding a taller stem, or swapping out your bars, brakes, and shifters entirely.

Mountain Bikes

Mountain bikes were at one time a fashionable choice for city riding, and the budgeting bike shopper is likely to encounter quite a few used ones. If you are less than 5'3" tall, the majority of suitable used bikes you'll find will likely be either vintage cruisers or mountain bikes with 26" wheels.

Mountain bikes can serve well enough as city bikes. They are, however, designed for riding on dirt and gravel roads and trails and single track in the wild, often up and down steep hills. Mountain bikes typically come with thick, knobby tires, which you will probably want to swap out for smoother and narrower ones to improve your speed on city streets. Most mountain bikes come with shocks, which cushion the ride. For city riding, avoid the kind with shocks in both the front and back ("full suspension"). If the shocks are only in the front fork, that doesn't need to be a deal-breaker—the fork can be readily switched with a non-bouncing one, or you may even want to keep it if your area is particularly plagued with pot holes.

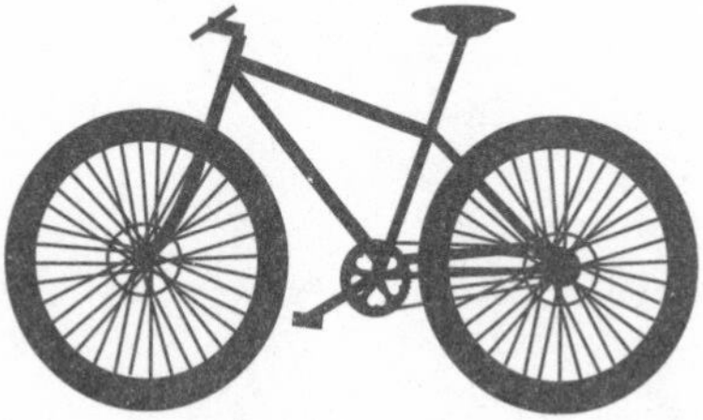

Mountain bike frame geometry is different from road bikes, and some people find them more comfortable. They generally come with straight-across handlebars rather than the drop bars of road bikes; you'll be more upright than when riding a road bike, but likely still positioned for more speed than a cruiser, Dutch bike, or hybrid. You may run into difficulties attaching racks and fenders to many mountain bikes. Many come with attachment points, but for others you will need to jury-rig a way to attach them, which is often not ideal, particularly for fenders.

Touring Bikes

A touring bike is similar to a road bike, but heavier and sturdier, with a frame design that makes them more comfortable for long, straight hauls. They tend to be suitably geared for hilly rides, and have the advantages of built-in attachment points for both front and rear racks. They will also take fenders without a struggle, and often have room for extra water bottle cages. All of these features can make them good everyday bikes.

Hybrids

Hybrids are what athletically oriented bike shops tend to keep in stock as "commuters." New hybrids are in the low to medium price range, and they are in fact often an excellent choice for your transportation needs, especially if you're just getting started. Hybrids are, as you may suspect, something in between a road bike and a mountain bike. They offer mountain-bike style handlebars and brakes, lots of gears, and a semi-upright posture, along with tires and frame geometry suitable for asphalt. They can be comfortably ridden for many miles at a time, though they will not carry you quite as fast as a road bike nor carry you comfortably down rutted mountain trails the way a mountain bike can. If you aren't sure what you're looking for in a bike, and are daunted by the options out there, a hybrid offers a reliable way to start riding.

Cruisers

There are two varieties of bicycle called cruisers, though they don't share much in common.

Modern cruisers are essentially beach bikes. They feature wide tires, a single speed, kick brakes (you pedal backwards to stop the bike), a wide, soft seat, and a frame geometry that puts you in a laid back posture. These bikes have snazzy paint jobs and are excellent for a mellow, flat ride down the boardwalk or the bike trail. They generally do not come with racks, but you can easily put a basket on the handlebars.

Vintage cruisers generally feature step-through frames, an upright sitting posture, three speeds, and heavy steel frames. They are not meant to travel quickly or far, but they are better suited to everyday urban riding than their modern counterparts. These usually do not come with racks, but they are likely to have fenders and a chain guard, and are practically begging to be outfitted with a front wire basket.

Comfort Bikes

So-called comfort bikes are marketed to people who fear that bicycling might not be for them. Unfortunately, this type of bike often successfully convinces them of that. Comfort bikes resemble hybrids, but with an even more upright posture and swept back handlebars. They come with exaggeratedly wide, cushioned seats, and most are equipped with shock-absorbing seat posts and forks, both of which look reassuring on the shop floor but increase the amount of effort required to ride. These bikes are fine for occasional jaunts down the bike path or boardwalk, but are not meant to be ridden any great distance or speed or while carrying cargo of any kind.

"Women's" Bikes

Occasionally a major bicycle manufacturer will decide to test the market for female bicycle buyers. You can spot these bikes a mile away by their easter egg color paint schemes and floral decals. They are built differently from these manufactures' other bikes, with dimensions based on several assumptions about fit: Namely, that women are smaller in stature than men, have narrower shoulders, smaller hands and feet, and proportionally longer legs and shorter torsos. These assumptions are by no means universally accurate, which is one reason why there are plenty of wide-shouldered women and long-legged men out there riding ill-fitting bicycles. Regardless, some shops will steer any female who walks through the door directly to their selection of "women's bikes." If your dimensions reflect the industry's equations, by all means, take a test ride—no matter what your gender.

Tricycles

People who are seeking extra balance and stability are often drawn to tricycles. But trikes are not necessarily easier to ride than two-wheelers. They are prone to tipping onto two wheels while you turn, and can be more difficult to ride in a straight line on a road with any sideways slope. Nonetheless, many people swear by tricycles, with recumbent trikes—which you can go quite fast on—having particularly fervent devotees.

The trick to keeping your tricycle upright is to lean in the opposite direction as you would on a two-wheeler—away from the direction of your turn, rather than into it.

Recumbents

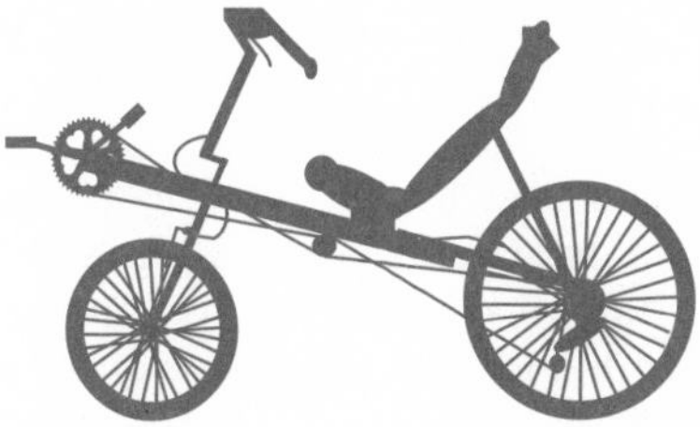

Recumbent bicycles, or 'bents, are something you either love or hate. On these bikes (or trikes), you sit in a little chair, leaning backwards. Your feet are on pedals in front of you, and your hands control the steering and brakes from your sides.

Recumbents are the domain of long distance riders and by the subset of the cycling population who cannot comfortably adjust to regular bike saddles. 'Bent riders are fans of being able to put their foot on the ground without dismounting at stops and the more laid back vantage point these bikes allow. There is quite a bit of fierce debate over the merits of recumbent riding; you're either a recumbent person or you aren't, it seems, and the only way to find out is to give it a try.

Handcycles

Hand-cranked tricycles, which are propelled with your hands and arms rather than your feet and legs, haven't yet made it into the cycling mainstream. They can be steered by anyone who wants to learn how, but they are currently mainly used among people with spinal cord injuries or disabilities that make a foot pedaled bike difficult to use. Nearly all handcycles have three wheels and are recumbents; they are primarily manufactured by the medical equipment industry and used for recreational purposes. There is a small but growing movement of people who are using non-recumbent handcycles (currently only bicycle manufacturer, Sun, produces these) for daily transportation in lieu of wheelchairs.

Folding Bikes

Folding bicycles are beloved by frequent travelers, tiny apartment dwellers, and people who combine bicycling with public transportation. The best folding bikes ride like full-sized bikes and have a small but wide range of gears. Some even have racks and lights built in. A dizzying array

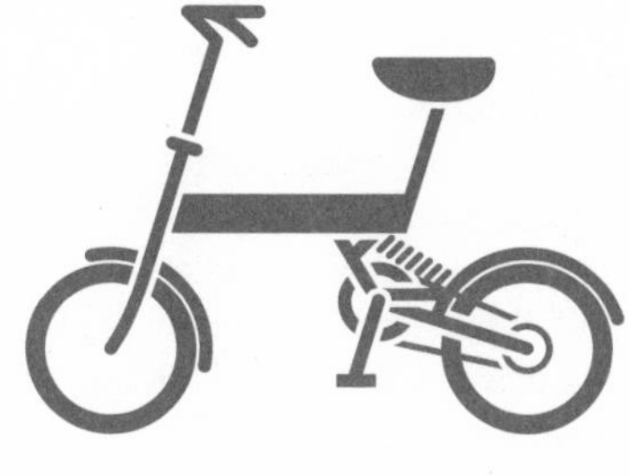

of options are available in terms of sturdiness, ease of folding, ride comfort, and cost.

Bike Share Bikes

If your city has a bike share system, you know what kind of bikes I mean: Big, heavy, slow, one-size fits all clunkers in various states of repair. Experienced cyclists look on these bikes in horror—until they try the system and get hooked. Not for the slow ride or the squeaky chains, but for the convenience of being able to swipe a card, grab a bike, and dock it again a couple of miles down the road without a care for the special bike clothes, locks, maintenance, storage, or theft concerns they may take for granted with their own faster, fancier steeds. A bike share bike is like having one more bicycle option than usual, there for you whenever you need a workhorse to get you to an appointment on time.

Cargo Bikes

"Spend big, expect lots." —*Joe Biel*

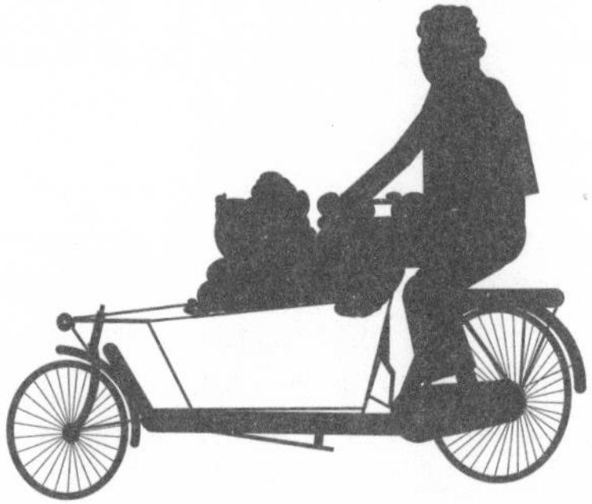

Cargo bikes tend to be heavy, but they can also carry more weight more comfortably than any other type of bike. If you have more to carry on a daily basis than can be comfortably hauled on your regular bike, a cargo bike might be right for you.

All cargo bikes will handle very differently with and without a load, which is worth keeping in mind when you are test-riding them. Chapter five has a more in-depth section on choosing and using cargo bikes, much of which remains applicable even if you are not carrying children.

Longtails

The longtail is the quintessential U.S. cargo bike. Nearly as narrow as a regular bicycle, these bike frames extend several feet longer in the back, with the rear wheel moved farther back. The bike's center of gravity is lower, allowing more stability overall. The result is that you can carry much larger and heavier items than on a regular-sized bike, keeping them centered over the rear wheel in side panniers.

Longtails were invented for the purpose of carrying two hundred pounds of green coffee beans along a mountainous dirt trail in Central America, or to carry sacks of grain down rutted roads in Rwanda. It turns out they work just as well for hauling a set of kitchen chairs, a month's worth of groceries, or two preadolescent children around a hilly U.S. city. They have been embraced as one of the most practical, fast, lightweight, and affordable cargo bike options available.

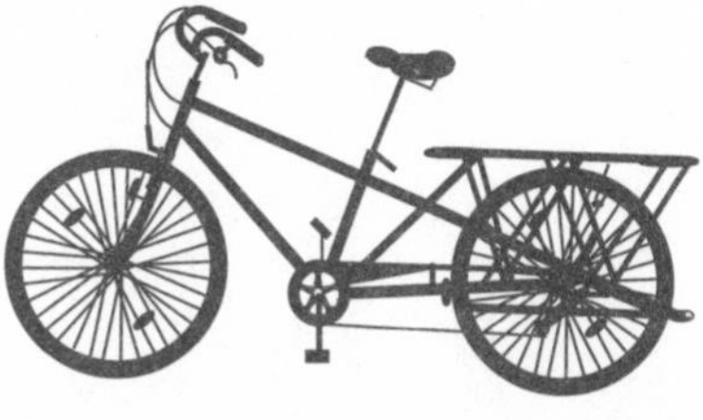

The variety of longtail options on the market is increasing rapidly. Xtracycle, the original company to introduce them, also makes a kit that can be used to convert your existing bicycle into a longtail. Whatever option you choose, a step-through frame is preferable, especially if you'll be carrying anything on the top deck of the longtail that might make it difficult to swing your leg over.

Frontloaders

Frontloader cargo bicycles are a different kind of bike altogether. They are a staple in the bicycle-friendly cities of Northern Europe. Recent years have seen a growing interest in them in the United States, particularly among families. The kind you are most likely to see in the U.S. is the Dutch "bakfiets" (pronounced bock-feets; the plural is "bakfietsen"), named for its signature wooden box. These bikes are stable, but they are heavy. They take some upper body strength to ride, and handle differently than regular bicycles.

Other frontloaders are on the market that are lighter and feel more like riding a regular bike, and yet others are designed specifically for carrying children (see chapter five). Some front-loading cargo tricycles can be found as well, including models that are made in North America. Your options are increasing rapidly.

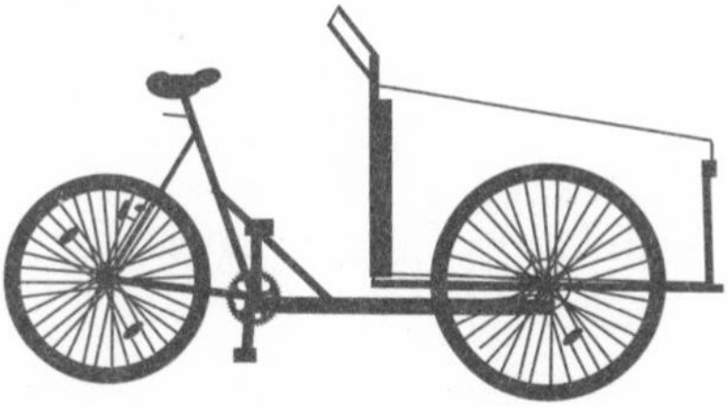

Bike Fit Basics

- When you sit on the saddle and hold the handlebars, with your feet horizontally even with each other on the pedals, your arms should be parallel to the angle of your thighs.

- Your hands should rest about shoulder width apart.

- You must be able to reach your brakes comfortably at all times, without reaching.

- Your weight should never be on your arms.

- Your seat should be high enough that your foot is flat on the pedal while your leg is nearly straight. It should not be so high that your legs are overextended or your hips rock side to side when you ride.

- The ball of your foot should rest on the center of the pedal.

- When you're standing over a diamond-frame bike with your feet on the ground, there should be at least a couple of inches between the top tube and your crotch.

Bike Fit

As a beginner, you don't need to know too much about bike fit. If you can easily reach both the pedals and the brakes and it doesn't hurt to ride, you're good to go. Have fun!

Most bike shop employees are trained in the basics of fitting and can help you choose a bike that is the right height and length for you. After that, adjusting the saddle position and handlebar tilt are often all that's needed to make your bike work. The trick to adjusting your bike fit is to do one type of adjustment at a time and only make incremental changes. Each centimeter can make a huge difference in the way your bike feels.

Professional Bike Fitting

If you end up riding many miles at a time, or racing, you may find you want to fine-tune the way your bike fits you. There's an art to this, and professional fitters exist who will, for a price, measure your dimensions and flexibility with lasers and computers and adjust your bike and its components to fit you down to the millimeter.

If you are having trouble finding a bicycle that feels comfortable, or if you have a body that the bike industry does not consider "standard," a professional fit is something to consider. A trained fitter will help you learn more about your body, your preferences, and what options are out there.

A Note on Custom, Handmade Bicycles

The next step up from a professional bike fit is having a bike made specifically to fit you.

There is a growing industry in the U.S. of custom, handmade bicycles, crafted and fit specifically to your body and needs. These bikes have the advantages of being beautiful, one-of-a-kind works of art as well as being made and built up with components to your exact specifications and measurements. They are manufactured by a skilled artisan and can sometimes take a year or more to build. As a result of these factors, custom bicycles cost thousands of dollars.

It is common for people who are new to bicycling to encounter difficulties with bike fit and quickly decide that they must have a custom bike. If you can afford this, then don't let me talk you out of it! But if it's a financial stretch, then I strongly encourage you to try other options first. As often as not, what you need to get comfortable is a minor saddle adjustment, a new handlebar set-up, or a bike that isn't too big for you. Even if your body is truly unusual, with one leg shorter than another, for instance, a clever modification in components will likely serve you better—and faster—than a whole new custom frame.

An investment in a handmade bicycle will suit you the best when you have a very specific and technically detailed idea of what you want from a bike. With custom bikes, you will get exactly what you ask for, and as a beginner you may not yet have the strongest sense of your exact needs. Once you are confident in your ability to choose and adjust an off-the-shelf bike to suit you, you'll be all the more ready to work with a frame builder to create the custom bicycle that will live up to all your wildest, highly developed fantasies.

Bikes for All Sizes

Many bike shop employees will try to steer bigger-bodied customers towards hybrids. That might be what you want—a slower, slightly more upright ride—but then again, it might not.

If you're heavy, that doesn't necessarily mean you need a special bike or components. If you're concerned about a bike being sturdy, look specifically at bikes made for utilitarian city riding, mountain bikes, and touring bikes—

they're built to get you up hills and take a beating. The weakest point on a bicycle is often the rear wheel, so if there's a lot of you (or if you habitually carry a lot of stuff on your bike) you may need to eventually get a stronger one. But don't let a bike shop employee talk you into this sort of thing until you've found that you actually need it.

Sadly, fat prejudice is alive and well in the bike industry. When bike shopping, it's extra important to find a shop where you feel comfortable and are treated with respect. If you run into problems, bring your business elsewhere.

Bikes for All Abilities

Bikes are a flexible medium, and can be adjusted to suit nearly every need. Once, while on a cross-country bike tour, a friend broke her right wrist. Instead of calling it quits, she had a local shop modify her bicycle so that she could operate both sets of brakes and shifters entirely with her left hand.

A vast array of options exists for what is called "adaptive cycling"—bicycle designs and styles that make human-powered transportation accessible to people with a wide range of abilities, injuries, and specific needs.

If you have impaired vision, many park systems have programs where you can ride on a tandem along with a sighted partner. If you can't count on having the strength on to pedal yourself everywhere and up every hill, go for more gears or an electric assist. If you can't pedal with your legs, try a handcycle. A national system of camps uses wide-tired bikes to teach kids with developmental disabilities to ride independently. Limitless variations exist on tandems, tricycles, and four wheelers. Some frame builders are working to build bicycle rickshaws that can accommodate wheelchairs. The bicycle variations out there are as brilliant and creative, as simple and complex, as the range of human needs and abilities.

More Considerations

Saddles

New riders are often tempted by saddles that are very wide and very soft, like cushy chairs. When you're pedaling, though, these enticing perches are often a recipe for discomfort.

In regards to width, your best option is a saddle that is wide enough to comfortably accommodate both of your sitz bones (the two bony protrusions you can feel where your inner thigh meets your crotch). There is considerable variation in this dimension between individuals, and it has nothing to do with your body type—you can have a large fundament and be most comfortable on a narrow saddle, or vice versa. If your saddle is too wide, the sides will chafe your legs when you pedal; if it is too narrow, you'll never find a comfortable seat.

As for softness, the myth is that a cushy, gel-filled saddle will shield your nether parts from chafing. Unfortunately, excess seat padding tends to have the opposite effect, creating more points of contact where painful chafing and saddle sores can occur. Everyone is different, but most people are happiest on a either lightly padded saddle or just hard leather that has been broken in over time to fit their shape. Many people prefer saddles with a cut out down the center (available in different variations for both men and women), while others find this feature painful. You may need to try different saddles (and different combinations of saddles and trousers and/or technical bike shorts) in order to find what's best for you. Some bike shops allow you to test ride seats—if yours does, take them up on it!

Your seat should be just high enough that your leg is straight when the ball of your foot rests on the pedal at its lowest point, but not so high that your leg locks or that you need to rock your hips back and forth to ride. You'll also want to move the saddle far enough forward that you can reach the brakes without locking your arms. If doing so puts your seat too far forward for comfort, then your bike is too long for you.

Saddle angle matters, too. If the saddle nose is irritating your crotch, it might make the most sense, counter-intuitively, to tip it upwards slightly—this pushes your weight further back, onto your butt. If you have the opposite problem, tip the saddle forward a bit—but not so far forward that your weight rests on your arms. If adjusting your saddle tilt doesn't improve matters, then return it to level and adjust your handlebar tilt instead.

Gears and Shifting

The gears on your bike amplify the power of your pedaling. If you need to get up a hill or get started with a heavy load, shifting down (that's to a smaller chain ring up front or a larger one in the back) will give you a boost. If you're cruising downhill or on the level and want to go faster, shifting up will transfer more of that power directly into making your wheels spin. Shift just before you begin to go uphill, and the chain will slide more smoothly onto the next gear. You must continue pedaling while you shift.

How many gears do you need? There are plenty of books out there that go into the topic in mathematical detail, if that interests you. It's actually pretty simple. If you live somewhere with hills, or plan to carry anything heavy on your bicycle, you'll be happier with more gears. If you'll be riding relatively flat streets without a lot of stuff, only one gear might be enough, three should be fine, and ten will certainly be adequate.

If you're on the fewer-gears end of the spectrum, you might want to spend some extra money on an internally geared hub (some vintage cruisers have these as well). These have several benefits. The gearing is protected from the weather and barely needs maintenance. While you cannot shift and pedal at the same time with these hubs, you do not have to remember to shift down before stopping while going uphill.

The Electric Assist, Demystified

An electric assist is like having a bunch of extra gears on your bike. It is fundamentally different from a motorized scooter or moped in that it has no throttle and can't power you up a hill while you sit back and relax. On an e-bike, you're unlikely to top 20mph even when it's maxed out. What it can do is help flatten that steep hill on the way home from the grocery store. If the hills are very steep and what you're carrying is very heavy, or if your body isn't up to the effort of whatever it is that you're doing, that's worth something.

Some cargo and family bike riders are starting to adopt electric assists. Other fans are people who live at the top of a steep hill, or need to avoid exertion for health reasons, or simply prefer to avoid getting sweaty on the way to work.

The downside to an electric assist is that it is expensive—between the assist unit and the battery, you can end up doubling or quadrupling the cost of your bike. The batteries can be bulky and heavy—meaning that if you run out of juice, or simply don't want to use the assist, you'll find yourself with one more big thing to haul. But technology is changing quickly, especially with the advent of electric assist units that are built into the rear bicycle wheel.

If you're curious about electric assists, it's worth taking a few out for test rides. But keep in mind that with enough gears on an unassisted bicycle, you may discover you have all the power you need.

Maintaining Your Bike

For many new riders, bike maintenance is a black box. But keeping your bike in working order can be as simple or as complex as you want it to be.

There is nothing wrong with handing your bike over to a shop every time anything seems a bit off, and this practice is in fact not as expensive as you might think. Likewise, spending a little extra on buying a bike that rarely needs to be maintained (and especially on tires that rarely have flats) is the best path for many. There are benefits to learning a few tricks yourself, though—as you'll discover the first time you realize you have a flat tire after your local shop is closed for the night.

In fact, nothing about bike maintenance is particularly difficult once you have learned how to do it. It doesn't take any special mechanical abilities—just some attention and a willingness to learn, one small step at a time.

You can hand over your bike to your trusty local bike shop and they'll fix what ails it, for a fee. That's a fine option and there is absolutely no shame in never, ever touching your bike with maintenance in mind. There are other ways to go, though, especially for simpler routine maintenance tasks like cleaning your chain and adjusting your brakes, intermediate ones like changing flat tires, and advanced bike wizardry like cleaning and repacking your hubs. I list a few bare bones upkeep tasks below that will extend the life of your bike and keep it out of the shop. If you want to learn more, there are many, many resources for learning everything you want to know about bikes and more.

Community Bike Projects

There's a different kind of bike shop proliferating in cities and towns around the world. They're called "community bike projects," "bike co-ops," or sometimes funny and whimsical names. You can usually identify them by the smiles and bustling atmosphere inside and the giant heaps of donated bike frames and parts out back.

These are places where anyone can go and get a bike, or bike repairs, or parts, or gear for free or very cheaply. Everything is donated, and most such shops are run entirely by volunteers. There's a catch, though: you'll need to do the work yourself, and you'll often need to trade volunteer hours for parts and frames.

Volunteers are on hand to guide you through fixing or building your bike, giving you tips and encouragement step by step as you diagnose your bike repair needs, find the parts, and take things apart and put them back together. It might sound intimidating, but the beauty of bicycling is that nearly everything is easily fixed and there are only a few simple systems to learn about. It's incredibly empowering and a great way to meet people and find out about other rides, events, and activism opportunities.

These bike projects often have a weekly or monthly night just for female and trans identified persons. Increasingly they're called WTF (which stands for women, trans, femme) or FTW (ditto, but the other way around) nights. If your local project doesn't have one, there's no reason you can't start one, even if your bike knowledge is rudimentary. These places are all about people from all different walks of life helping each other make things happen.

Be Your Own Mechanic

If it's more your style to figure things out for yourself in the privacy of your home, why not learn to be your own mechanic? All you need is some elbow grease, patience, time, and a good book or access to the internet, where you can find words, photos, and videos to help you learn to do any bike maintenance task you can dream of. See EverydayBicycling.com for some specific resources.

Basic Tips

Here are some extremely basic tips to start you out:

• **Air up.** Tires need the air topped off occasionally; more often in the summer. Buy a floor pump for this purpose or swing by a bike shop occasionally to use theirs. The little portable pumps that you can throw in your bag for emergencies are annoying to use and won't get your tires up to full pressure.

Each tire has a recommended range of pounds of pressure—measured in pounds per square inch, or PSI—that's written right on the sidewall. Most tires have a recommended pressure range. Try to keep it within five or ten pounds of the maximum. If you over-inflate your tires, you'll notice you'll start to send chunks of gravel flying. If you under-inflate them, you'll have to work a lot harder to ride, and you risk the dreaded pinch flat or snakebite from your tube getting pinched between the tire and the wall of the rim.

• **Flat tires** are the most common maintenance problem you'll have. A time will come when you'll be riding along and hear either a loud pop or a slow hiss, and suddenly you'll have a puncture. Actually, they're a bit of a misnomer. While it's possible for the tire itself—the part that comes into contact with the ground—to wear through or develop a hole in it, most flats are actually caused by punctures in the much thinner rubber tube that sits inside the tire.

Most flats are caused either by a piece of glass embedded in your tire that's worked its way through to the tube or else by the tube being pinched between the tire wall and the rim when the air pressure gets too low. Patching or replacing the tube is usually quick and not very expensive if a bike shop does it; it's even cheaper if you learn to do it yourself.

• **Keep your chain clean.** All you need is a rag and a little bottle of chain lube (definitely don't use anything but made-for-the-purpose chain lube unless you're in a real pinch). Flip your bike upside-down, wipe the gunk off your chain and gears, put a drop of lube on each link, spin the pedals a few times to work it all in, and then wipe off all the lube. Voila. If the weather's wet, you might even do this every day. This will keep your gears from wearing out prematurely—they're expensive to replace, so this basic maintenance helps your pocketbook as well as your ability to shift.

• **Brakes and rims.** The more you brake, the more your brake pads wear down. As this happens, they leave a layer of debris on the metal rims of your wheels. When your rims are dirty, they wear your brake pads down even faster, like sandpaper. It's a good idea to get in the habit of wiping down the rims with a (non-greasy) rag every week or so, and more often in wet weather. Also keep an eye on your brake pads. When they are down to the wear line, have them replaced. If you let them go further, you won't be able to brake easily; and if you let them wear down to the metal, they'll tear up your rims. This is another piece of cost-effective maintenance, as wheels are a lot more expensive to replace than brake pads.

• **The annual checkup.** It's in the nature of screws to come unscrewed, especially as you ride for months over bumpy roads. Brake pads wear down and so do chain rings. Rubber gets old and needs to be replaced. Cables wear out. Hubs need to be adjusted. Derailleurs can get finicky. It's a good idea to bring your bike into a shop for an annual once-over, preferably at either the end of winter or the beginning, or both. Or do an annual checkup yourself, working through the chapters of a bike maintenance book.

Protect Your Bike

In any city, a good lock is a necessity. Lock your bike up any time you leave it alone—on a city street, in your own backyard or garage, or in your house while you're on vacation. Cable locks, however burly, will not do you any good—they can be snipped with shears in seconds. Spend a bit more and get a u-lock. These make your bike so difficult to steal that some brands come with insurance.

How you lock your bike matters as well. A designated bike parking staple or rack is probably your best bet, so long as it's securely bolted to the ground. A street sign is usually safe as well, though if bike theft is rampant in your city, make sure the sign at the top, no matter how high, is wide enough that your lock can't be slid over it, and that the sign is bolted firmly into concrete.

Always lock your bike through the frame and around an immovable object. If your u-lock is big enough, also capture one of your wheels within the lock; wheels are an easy target for thieves. Your front wheel is easier for an opportunist to remove, but rear wheels are more valuable (and expensive to replace). Which wheel you lock is up to you; in very high-theft cities, carry two u-locks so you don't have to choose.

Before your bike ever has a chance to be stolen, write down its serial number. This will be necessary to prove ownership in case it shows up at a pawnshop or is turned in to the police. The serial number is usually etched on the bottom bracket, below where the pedals attach to the bike. Take a photo of yourself and your bike and write the serial number on the back; or email yourself a digital photo and serial number with enough descriptive text that you can easily search for it again.

If your bike is stolen, alert the police. There are also several services on the Internet for registering stolen bikes, and there is a reasonable chance that searching online merchants that sell used bikes might turn up yours. If you don't find it again, your lock manufacturer, homeowner's insurance, or renter's insurance may cover the loss.

4

CARRYING THINGS BY BIKE

"Experiment, don't give up, lash it down good, go slow." —*Sara Stout, Portland*

When I first started riding a bike, I slung my purse strap across my chest, hopped on, and rode off. I soon graduated to putting the purse in a rickety metal front basket. This was my first bicycle accessory and the most revelatory by far until my discovery, years later, of the rear rack.

My front basket meant speed and freedom. Suddenly I could return my library books on the way to work and pick up a load of groceries afterwards without worrying about marring my professional outfit with a backpack. I could run spontaneous errands and bring leftovers home from a restaurant. In a city built for cars, I suddenly had a taste of how daily life could be not only functional without one, but easier and more flexible.

In the decade since then I've carried a lot of things on my bikes, and done it a lot of different ways. There's no better feeling than arriving across town with your unlikely load intact, be it cupcakes or lumber. I've had my share of misadventures too, and hopefully this chapter will save you from repeating some of them. You learn, over time, to double check that your bungie cords are tight. You also learn that when you apply your brain to the task of carrying something by bicycle, there's very little you can't bring with you.

Wearing Your Cargo

The simplest way to carry something on your bike is often the same way you would carry it off the bicycle. Put your keys in your pocket, sling your shoulder bag across your chest, tie your sweater around your waist. So long as you keep things close to your body and out of the spokes, you'll often be fine even if you have no other carrying capacity.

You'll find yourself pushing the limits of this method, though, the first time you find yourself trying to ride home with a full grocery bag swinging from your handlebars, banging against the spokes, upsetting your balance, and threatening to send you toppling into the curb.

This scenario tends to lead people quickly to the backpack or messenger bag. Both are easy, noncommittal solutions, requiring no hardware or adjustments to your bike and allowing you to get on and off your bike with minimal hassle. You'll find the bag just as useful when you don't have your bike with you. In fact, you probably already own something like this.

Messenger bags sport a single strap that runs across your chest and over one shoulder. They get their name from their origins among bike messengers who require the convenience of being able to swivel their bag around their body for quick access to the packages inside as they run in and out of an office.

If you don't need easy, constant access to your bag as you ride around, you'll find a backpack to be just as convenient. A backpack is also far kinder to your back and neck, particularly if you often carry heavy items. Whatever you use, you'll be most comfortable with the bag strapped tightly to your body, maybe with a waist strap, and with the weight higher rather than lower.

For bicycling, look for a backpack or bag that is waterproof. If the one you use doesn't keep water out well, stow a plastic trashbag in an easy to access compartment to protect your stuff in case you're caught in a downpour.

Less is often more; and it's a universal truth that the more carrying capacity you have, the more you will find to carry. Sometimes it's nice to travel light, and at these times an excellent way to carry your essentials is a hip pouch. This does not need to resemble the fanny pack of yesteryear if that isn't your style. Several small companies make attractive, waterproof hip pouches specifically with bicycling in mind. Some are made with a slot to handily carry your u-lock while you ride.

Letting the Bike Do the Work

Carrying your belongings on your back has its advantages, but also its downsides. Backpacks make your back sweaty in the summer, and the weight, besides being ergonomically awkward, can lead to injuries.

The good news is that your bicycle can comfortably carry the same load as your back, and then some. Unfortunately, most bikes in North America are still sold without carrying capacity, and adding it is often up to you. Fortunately, there are many options out there.

The Front Basket

The front basket is iconic and for a reason.

A basket provides easy access to your things. You won't need to get off your bike or awkwardly rummage through your shoulder bag when you ride up to the drive-through window at the bank or pause to have a snack. You can quickly grab your camera, and no effort is needed to get out your pen to jot down the phone number of the friend you've just run into.

The flimsy woven plastic basket with the plastic flower that graced your bike as a kid might not hold up under the loads you carry today. But a small wicker basket to throw your purse or wallet and keys into is still one of the handiest bike accessories available. Large, sturdy metal baskets are also available, and tend to be quite affordable.

Baskets usually mount to your handlebars. This means that if you ride a road bike with drop bars, the kind that curve forward, a basket might not be your best option, though a handlebar bag might work well. Larger baskets have struts that can be attached to your fork, increasing their load bearing capacity.

A word of caution: if you hit a big enough pothole at a high enough speed, the contents of your front basket will fly up and out, possibly hitting you in the face, possibly breaking all over the road. So if you ride at more than a leisurely pace, some kind of cover is a good idea, or even just a bungie cord or two to keep the contents inside. Also be watchful for any straps dangling through the holes of your basket that might get caught in your front wheel.

Cargo Up Front

A basket is convenient for small things. But what if you want to carry more weight? While many people prefer to put their weight over their rear wheel, there is a strong faction, including many long distance bike tourers, that prefers to carry their load up front. How you distribute the weight on your bicycle affects how it feels to ride; the choice is a personal one, though some bikes are engineered to be most comfortable carrying the load up front.

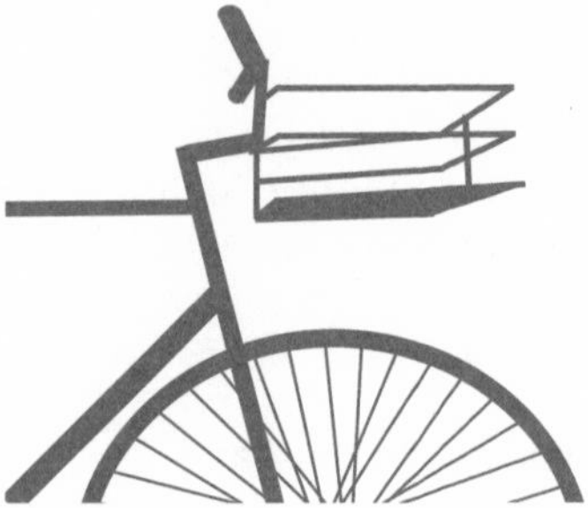

The classic way to carry a lot of weight in the front is a front rack that sits low and center over the wheel. The racks consist of bars on which you can hang small panniers. Another option is the porteur rack, a shelf that sits over your front wheel and can serve as the base for a large-ish, boxy bag of the type that is beloved by long-distance cyclists.

Another option is more difficult to find and also more expensive, though quite sturdy. This is the rack or platform that attaches to the bicycle frame itself rather than the handlebars. This type of rack allows you to carry very heavy loads in a way that does not affect your steering. When you turn the handlebars, the rack doesn't move, making for a smoother, more stable ride.

The Rear Rack

My first rear rack, once I finally got it installed, changed everything for me. I kept a couple of bungie cords strapped to it at all times and used them to hold down whatever I needed to carry: a stack of books, my backpack, a load of groceries, a chair found at the side of the road. This is a strategy that can get you through many years and many quandaries gracefully and happily.

If your bike doesn't already have a rear rack on it, get one. If you have one, use it! You'll be amazed at what it can carry. But use a couple of bungie cords and reasonable caution when you turn, and it also isn't that difficult.

Racks run from very cheap to very spendy. Most bike shops should have at least one basic, $25 model on hand and can attach it to your bike for a small fee. Most racks feature a platform of sorts on top, a bar on each side to hang panniers from, and protrusions near the axle to hook your pannier or bungie cord onto from below. Some racks have

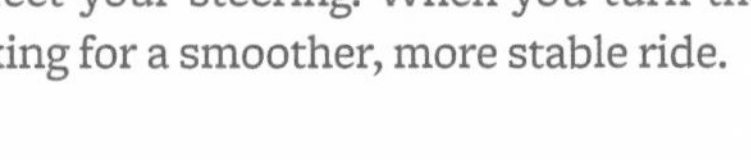

holes punched in the back where you can mount a permanent, relatively theft proof, red light.

Installing racks yourself can be a drag. Chances are your bike is not an exact match for the prototype any given rack was designed for. Unless this is the sort of task you love, it can be well worth paying your mechanic to do it for you.

If you carry a lot of weight, you'll need to think about bike maintenance slightly more often than otherwise. Keep an eye on your brake pads—they're working harder and will wear out faster. Also be mindful of your wheels, especially your rear one—if you see any bent or broken spokes, replace them right away, or better yet invest in a stronger wheel.

Bungies and Tie-Downs

Bungie cords are inexpensive new, but if you're really on a budget there are better options. Once you've patched an inner tube more than a few times or suffered a major blowout, it can take on a new, useful life as a tie-down. Some people cut out the valve and tie simple knots or loops. Others leave it intact, wrapping it around their load and rack. Aside from being free—and freely available in bulk at any bike shop—the distinct advantage over a bungee cord is that you don't have a high-stress elastic cord with metal hooks on the end that can seriously injure you.

Whatever you use, strap your cargo down very tightly, with the elastic stretched to its fullest. Believe that whatever you are carrying will use all its wiles to escape, and stay a step ahead of it.

You can use just about anything in a pinch, from your scarf to your sweater to a piece of butcher's twine or ribbon scrounged up by a supermarket employee. Use your shoelaces if you need to. Whatever you use, pull it taut and triple check the stability of your load before you set off.

If you use bungies with metal hooks, don't let them snap back and take out your eyeball. Also, make sure you keep everything out of your spokes, from tie-downs that aren't in use to your long skirt or scarf to your pants leg. Extracting a bungie from your hub is not fun. Being stopped short while in traffic by a hooked spoke can be disastrous, particularly if it is your front wheel that is hooked. Be especially careful to keep all tie downs and straps from dangling anywhere near your wheels.

Rear Baskets

My next revelatory upgrade was the twenty-dollar folding basket that mounted to one side of the rear rack. The purchase was inspired by an artist friend who had two of these and could regularly be seen trucking around town with her silkscreened tote bag containing wallet and keys in one basket and a grocery bag or stack of letterpress greeting cards in the other. In the rain, she put everything in plastic bags.

As with a front basket, a rear basket is wonderfully convenient. You can just put your backpack, a stack of books, a diaper bag, or a recent purchase in these and ride off. The baskets fold up, which is good if you keep your bike in a narrow hallway. These rear baskets are not extremely durable and are often difficult to mount to your bike. But overall they work great, are a good value, and are about as basic as it gets.

Crates

A time-honored carrying technique is a plastic crate on your rear rack, the type that milk bottles come in. These are found in various shapes, sizes and colors; you probably already have one in your basement, maybe holding records. Attach it to your rack with hose clamps from the hardware store or for a more removable option, strap it on tight with bungie cords.

Panniers

Panniers are saddlebags; they're like backpacks for your bicycle, usually detachable, that hang from the side of a front or rear rack.

The iconic city cycling panniers are made by the German company Ortlieb. Their distinctive design is based on rafting bags meant to withstand prolonged submersion. The basic model is just a heavy-duty waterproof bag that rolls down and clips on the top. Plastic clips on the side hook over the top of your rear rack, and a bracket at the bottom keeps the bag from rattling or falling outwards as you turn. They come in bold, bright colors with reflectors on the sides. They're spendy but they last.

Multiple companies now make similar bags, and many have expanded on this basic design with welcome features like external and internal pockets (essential if you ever want to find your house keys or wallet when you need them), and a waterproof hood that stretches over the top of the bag.

Make Your Own Bike Buckets!

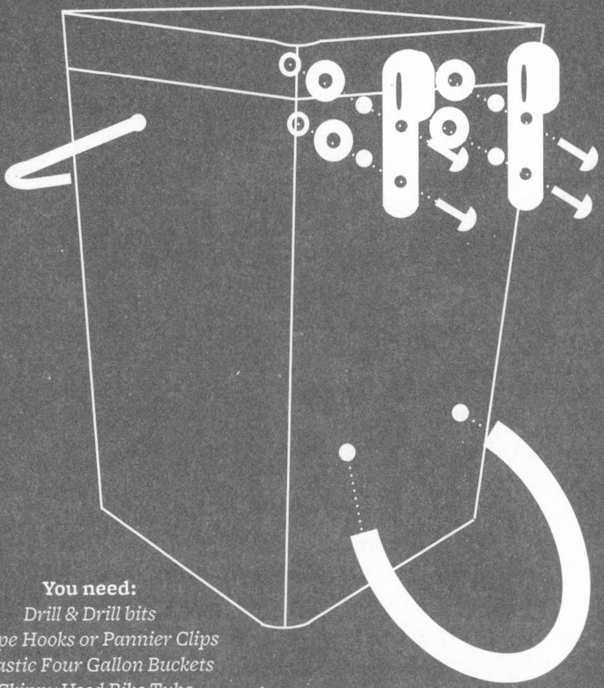

You need:

Drill & Drill bits
4 Rope Hooks or Pannier Clips
2 Plastic Four Gallon Buckets
1 Skinny Used Bike Tube
Scissors
8 Nuts, Bolts, and Washers
Screwdriver

1. Position your bucket so the top sits level with your bike rack without the bottom disturbing your derailleur.
2. Measure, mark, and drill holes (six black holes) so the inner tube will stretch taut when on your bike.
3. Pull the tube through the holes on the bottom and tie knots on each end inside the bucket
4.Bolt your clips or rope hooks in.
5. Attach to your bike rack and test it by riding around the block.

The downside of panniers is that when you get off the bike you must lug them around by their finger-wrenching handle or spine-twisting shoulder strap. This is not a big deal unless you are carrying a lot of weight—a laptop computer, some books, a double load of groceries. If you spend a lot of time walking with all your things in between getting on and off the bike, you may be happier with a backpack and basket combination.

You might also run across touring panniers. These are not always waterproof, and have a great number of internal and external pockets. They feature rugged hardware and—of course—nowhere to clip a shoulder strap.

Sometimes people will use a cable lock to keep their panniers attached to their bike; they just have their stuff in another, more walking-friendly bag inside the pannier. This is a good option if you live in a place where you don't worry about the cable or strap being cut and the pannier disappearing. Transverse panniers—a staple Dutch bicycle accessory that permanently attaches to your rack—are great for this. You can also purchase square pannier-baskets that are shaped to fit a single grocery bag and intended to be left on the bicycle in low-theft areas.

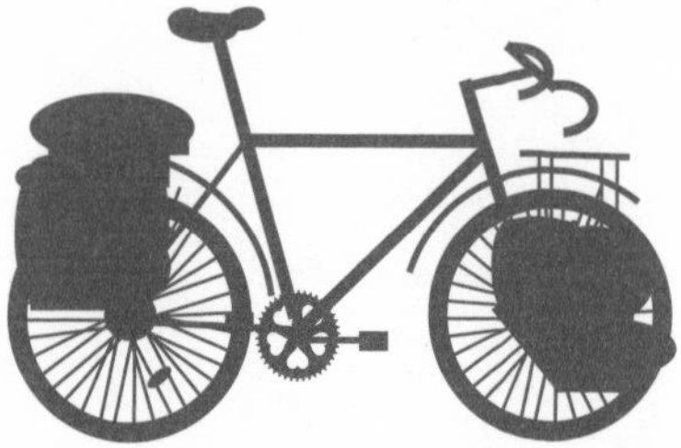

A somewhat dizzying array of panniers is now becoming available that more closely resemble fashionable purses and briefcases, or conversely that are made of oilcloth and suitable for rugged outdoor use. These are all very different in their attachments and closures as well as their aesthetics. When choosing a pannier for daily use, a primary consideration should be how easily it can be easily opened, closed, and taken on and off the bike multiple times a day.

A Note About Kickstands

Aside from a rack, the one investment that will instantly improve the way your bike works for you is the kickstand. For under ten dollars and less than five minutes spent fiddling with a wrench, the kickstand will change your life. No more returning to the sign you've locked your bike to only to find it lying helpless on the ground. No more awkwardly holding your bike one-handed while struggling into your rain pants mid-commute.

There are two kinds of kickstands: the most common one mounts onto your bottom bracket—the part of your frame that's between your pedals. This is fine for light use—picking up a few groceries, or taking your laptop to work or your books to school.

A sturdier option is the load-bearing kickstand that mounts to the rear triangle on the left side of your bike. This will keep your bike upright even though you've just balanced a box full of books from the library sale on your rear rack.

Yet burlier is the double kickstand. It costs more but will further revolutionize your life. This kickstand sits at your bottom bracket; when engaged it lifts your rear wheel off the ground and creates a tripod between its two prongs and your front wheel. This is an essential investment for cargo bikes and anyone carrying children. It's also handy for fixing flats on the fly. Triple kickstands exist as well.

Trailers

If putting racks on your bike is proving troublesome, or if you want to have the option to carry bulkier items than your racks can handle, a trailer is an excellent option.

Trailers are easy. You hitch them on, load them down, and ride off, feeling stable and only slightly more encumbered than before. When you're pulling the trailer, slow down on turns. Take it easy on hills. And remember that you're longer than you used to be.

Kid Trailer

Trailers built for carrying children have a distinctive upright shape, cloth seats and basic seatbelts inside, and an aluminum frame with a roll bar surrounded by a cloth cover; some have a clear plastic "window" at the top that rolls up to let air in through a mesh screen. For carrying actual kids (or your dog), see chapter five.

For carrying cargo, a used kids trailer is usually a good, cheap bet, with little to no modification needed. They have the added benefit of inspiring anyone driving past you to give you a bit of extra room.

These trailers are abundant, gathering dust in garages all across the country as their original passengers outgrow them. In most places you should be able to find a used model for $25 to $100, depending on its condition and demand, at a yard sale or online. Look for one with wheels that don't wobble, screws that can be tightened, inflatable tires, and exterior fabric that's in good enough condition to keep the elements off your stuff. In order for the trailer to be useful, the hitch needs to be in working order.

Modification possibilities are endless. You can maximize your capacity by removing the seat. Some people remove the fabric and make a new bottom out of a sheet of plywood cut to fit. A giant plastic tub can keep your belongings out of the elements.

Cargo Trailers

There's a blossoming of cargo trailers on the market, new and used, high end and low. You'll pay $300 to $500 for most new ones; it's possible to find cheaper ones, but you'll sacrifice sturdiness and durability.

For light, everyday uses, like weekend camping trips or stocking up on bulk flour and peanut butter, a lightweight, fabric-sided trailer should be fine. But be cautious when shopping: some lower end (though not necessarily cheaper ones) are held together with plastic parts, reducing their weight limit significantly.

If you'll be carrying heavier things, even occasionally—furniture shopping, helping out on bike moves, cleaning out your garage or bookshelves, bulk grocery shopping for the neighborhood, carrying an adult sitting on a stool playing the banjo, or the hundreds of occasions that come up over the course of a year that might otherwise send you straight to your local car-sharing service's sign up page—get something a little sturdier.

A workhorse trailer will have a wood or metal floor, and should have all metal attachments. Some kinds come with full sized bicycle wheels; others feature metal guards above the wheels for more easily carrying wide loads. Other trailers are long and trussed like a bridge, able to carry hundreds of pounds.

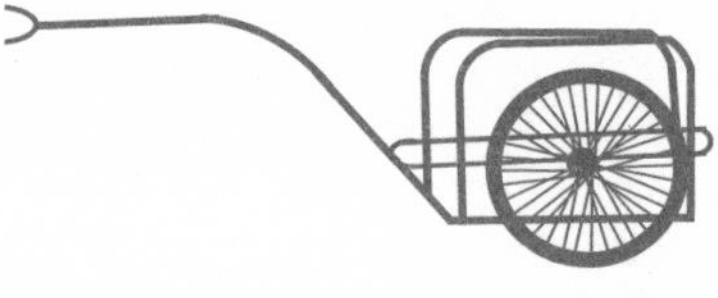

Most trailers have two wheels, but a few have a single wheel. These are small, light weight and don't take up much storage space. Not everyone likes the way they feel to ride with, and you must use caution and slow down when turning.

The Trailer Hitch

Before choosing a trailer, make sure it has a hitch that plays well with your bicycle.

On many cheaper trailers, the hitch is a hard plastic clamp that attaches to the rear left triangle of your bike frame or seatpost. This is easy to put on and remove, but does not hold up well under very heavy loads; also, some bicycles have design elements that are not compatible, and some racks and kickstands may also prevent you from using this hitch.

Sturdier, though less convenient, is the hitch that is attached to your rear hub. You can remove and attach the trailer easily, but must remove the wheel to move the hitch to another bicycle. This type of hitch places quite a bit of strain on your wheel; keep an eye out for bent or broken spokes as a sign you need to upgrade to a stronger wheel.

Some hitches attach to your bicycle's seat post, and are very functional unless you have a particularly short bicycle or if it interferes with carrying items on your rear rack. A seat post hitch is good for heavy loads, but make sure your trailer is loaded evenly side-to-side and front to back as it will pull on your bike. Balance is everything.

Extra Awesome Cargo Tactics

Carrying Heavy Things

Whenever you're carrying an unusually heavy load, it will feel wobbly at first, and you may wonder how you will manage it. Your body will learn the trick of stabilizing it quickly, though—it tends to take five or ten minutes to adjust. The faster you go, the smoother your ride will feel. Stopping and starting again will be the most difficult part, so if you need to carry something difficult, plan your route accordingly.

The best way to carry weight is low and centered over the wheel. If your weight is too far back or forward it will make your bike squirrely to handle. Some swear that heavier loads are easier to carry up front.

If a lot of your bicycling involves carrying heavy stuff, seriously look into investing in a cargo bike or tricycle. See chapter three for a rundown of your options.

Carrying Fragile Things

"It's impossible to not jostle something when it's strapped down, no matter how careful you are. I've carried many fancy cupcakes on bikes, both successfully and unsuccessfully. The successful times, I've had a canvas tote bag with a flat bottom that is big enough for the cupcakes container to sit level. You'll need to hold the bag or hang it from your handlebars so it can swing lightly. Swinging lightly is key, strapping down is what causes problems." —*Miriam R.*

Remember the exercise you did in grade school where you packaged up an egg and dropped it off the school roof? You'll have a similar challenge next time you buy eggs at the grocery store. Or when you offer to bake a cake for a friend's birthday. Or when you take a leisurely summer cruise out to your favorite berry patch and then want to get your seven pounds of blueberries home in berry rather than juice form. Or when you try to bring home a bouquet of flowers for your sweetie.

One danger to fragile items is simply getting jostled around in your bag when you ride over potholes or tilt to turn a corner. Eggs and light bulbs will survive just fine so long as they are put away compactly, so that they aren't free to rattle around and knock into other items in your bag. Soft fruit like bananas, on the other hand, should be packed no less snugly but should be surrounded by something that won't bruise it, like a bag of lettuce or a sweater.

The other peril fragile items face is road vibration. In the case of berries or flowers, your body is often going to be your best shock absorber.

Anything that can't be stabilized on all its surfaces, like a cake, will be better off firmly stuck to a plate that's in a plate-sized box that's cushioned with a blanket and sitting in your trailer or on your rack as you ride extremely slowly and carefully over the shortest distance possible. You can eke out a little extra shock absorption by letting some air out of your tires.

Your Beverage

It's always nice to have water around when you ride, and when you are going any distance and speed in hot weather, water becomes essential.

Many bikes come with a water bottle cage, or mounts to attach one. These are cheap to buy and easy to install. They are designed to hold the type of soft plastic water bottles you can buy at bike shops. Some water bottle cages—the bulky plastic ones—can hold a metal water bottle, though these have a tendency to pop out and roll across the road at inopportune moments. You might be better off with your hard plastic, metal, or glass beverage container in a pannier, perhaps one that's partly unzipped where the bottle can easily be reached at stop lights.

If you like to carry your coffee or tea with you while you ride, it's possible to purchase a bicycle-specific cup holder that attaches to your handlebars and holds a tapered cup conveniently close at hand. With a little ingenuity, you could also make your own.

Carrying Other Bicycles

The time-honored method for carrying a second bicycle is ghost riding. While riding one bicycle, you carefully guide the other bike along by grasping its stem (that's the part that attaches the handlebars to the frame). This requires some mojo and upper body strength. It's best to keep the second bike to your left so that your right hand is by your own rear brake; that way if you have to stop suddenly you won't fly over the handlebars.

If you have an Xtracycle, you're in luck—its panniers were designed with this need in mind. Strap the front wheel of the bike you're towing into the pannier (tightly!); the rear wheel rolls behind you.

Instructions abound on the Internet for making a DIY tow hitch for the rear rack of any bicycle. You remove the front wheel of the bike to be towed, drop the slots on the fork onto the hitch, strap the wheel to your pannier or back, and ride off.

If you have a trailer or cargo bike, you have two options. One is to take the wheels off the second bike and lash it down as well as you can. If bicycles were people, they'd be all elbows and knees, and it can take some finagling to keep the drive train away from your trailer wheel and prevent a rogue handlebar from scraping the ground. If you have the space, it's easiest to stand the bicycle upright on its two wheels, as though it were about to ride off, and lash it down tightly in that position.

How to Move by Bike

To the uninitiated, moving house by bicycle sounds barely believable. Those who have participated in a bike move know the truth—it's faster, easier, cheaper, and more fun than moving with a rented truck and a couple of strong friends.

A bike move is a social event. It's a barn raising, a housewarming party, and a parade all wrapped into one. Numbers are what make it work. When you have fifteen friends carrying your belongings out to their bikes, strapping down their loads, and then bringing everything inside at the destination, a move suddenly becomes efficient. It may take a bit longer to ride to your destination, but you save a huge amount of time and energy when you don't have to make twenty trips on each end to carry all your boxes to and from a truck.

The best way to learn the ways of the bike move is to participate in someone else's. If you're a pioneer, here are some tips to get you started:

1. Set a date and invite people. Do this at least a couple of weeks in advance, and remind people again a day or two before the move. If you're comfortable with friendly strangers helping out, promote it widely in your local bicycling scene. Plan it like it's a party. And it really is a party on wheels—you may have to make this clear in the invitation.

2. Have all your packing done by the day of the move. Loading everything up should take about an hour. Be sure to label anything that shouldn't be moved.

3. Food is key. Provide coffee and donuts at the beginning of the move, and beer and pizza at the end.

4. Plan your route in advance. Avoid steep hills and high-traffic streets as much as possible. Try to ride the route the day before your move to make sure there are no construction detours.

5. Have extra bungie cords and tie-downs on hand. If there's a chance of rain, provide tarps.

6. Plan ahead for the big items. Take an inventory of large items like beds and refrigerators and try to make sure enough friends with large bike trailers are able to be on hand. It's cool if you need to borrow someone's truck to finish the job, but don't underestimate the ingenuity of your movers.

7. Take pictures and share them online! The more people move by bike, the more people will want to move by bike...

Pets

The idea of getting around primarily by bike stalls, for many, when it comes to pets. Taking the dog to the park, the cat to the vet, or simply buying kitty litter are all issues that I've seen stymie even those who are most devoted to their bicycle way of life. Here are some ways I've gleaned from my own experiences and those of carfree friends.

I've heard tales of a parrot that goes bike touring along with its human, commenting on the scenery from its perch on her handlebars. But for the sake of this chapter I'm going to stick with advising you about what I know: dogs and cats.

Dogs

Running Alongside

Bicycling alongside your running dog requires a lot of trust between the two of you. It might not be the best idea if your dog is easily distractible or still learning to listen to you. But if your dog needs a lot of exercise and you can't keep up running with it, and if a good network of low-traffic streets is available, this might be the best of both worlds.

Unless you have an impeccably trained dog and live somewhere rural, it's a good idea to have the dog on a leash. This leads to the second problem of running with dogs, which is that they can get excited and run in front of your bike or into your spokes. To address this, there are gizmos you can purchase that are basically a short leash on a stick. The stick end attaches to your bike and is of a length to make sure the dog maintains a safe distance; the leash end attaches to the dog's harness and gives it enough leeway to run freely but not too freely.

On Your Bike or In a Trailer

I've seen a huge range of inventive setups for carrying your dog by bike. The easiest is simply putting your dog in any old trailer (or flatbed cargo bike) and securing it by short leash so that it can't jump out. A small dog can be carried in a basket or a bag. There are also dog-specific trailers that you can purchase in various sizes that come with ample mesh and plastic window options to let the smells in and the keep the elements out. I met a man once who had fashioned a custom trailer with a sturdy canvas wall to separate his two Corgies who could not get along in the same confined space.

Many dogs can hop right in a bike trailer for the first time and feel right at home, happily lolling their tongue as you cruise along. Unfortunately, many other dogs will be extremely nervous and suspicious of bicycle riding at first.

The trick to training your dog to love the bike is the same as with any sort of new skill or environment: Incremental steps and tons of rewards and praise. The idea is to go slowly and to use the dog's favorite things to create positive associations with each new level of involvement with the bike and trailer. Maybe immediately or maybe after much positive reinforcement, your dog will be ready to jump on board and go for a ride.

Cats

When I lived with someone who had a car, I used to dread having to take our cats to the vet. It was always the same scene: They hid, they resisted capture, they clawed desperately, contorting their bodies to shapes incompatible with the carrier door. Finally, scratched, late, and frustrated, I would haul the cage out to the car and try to tune out the piteous, trapped mewling that punctuated the entire drive.

Two years ago, when I first transported my cat by bike, I was prepared for exactly the same scene. I had wised up a bit, so instead of pulling the cat carrier out of the basement five minutes before it was time to go I brought it up a few days early, put a blanket and one of my sweatshirts in it, and left the door open. When it was time to go, I waved a treat enticingly under the cat's nose and he obligingly followed right into the cage, where he stared at me reproachfully from behind the door that I snapped shut behind him.

I brought the cage out to my longtail Xtracycle and strapped it into the side pannier, more or less level. Then we set out. I rode slowly on a back route, avoiding bumps. And something amazing happened—or rather, it didn't happen. The cat didn't cry. He didn't even look that upset. He just stared—and smelled—intently out from his carrier at the passing scenery, nearly at his normal eye level. When we got to the vet's office, they were impressed by how relaxed he was. Bikes might be the best thing for cats after all.

You don't need a longtail to carry your cat. If you've got a cat carrier, you can also place it in a trailer, strap it to the rear rack of your bike (if the carrier is small enough), or set it on the front platform of a front loading cargo bike.

Pet Food and Litter

Figuring out how to bring your actual pet along by bike is one thing; bringing home a huge bag of food or litter every couple of weeks is another. If you buy pet supplies by the giant bagful, you might be able to simply bungie it to your rack, arranging it so that the weight drapes about equally over each side. In a rainy climate, a carefully arranged trash bag will help prevent you from leaving a trail of kibble behind you.

If the rack solution proves cumbersome, investing in a bike trailer or a cargo bike may prove the way to go, and will greatly expand your options for buying other things in bulk as well.

Adult Passengers

A lot of people have a pretty common transportation need that often seems to preclude biking: Transporting other adults who may not have a bike or be able to ride themselves. That can mean anything from picking up your date for dinner when their bike has a flat tire to taking your elderly uncle to a doctor's appointment to traveling a few blocks with a friend who met you by car but doesn't want to lose their parking space. All these things can be accomplished by bicycle, if both parties are willing.

When my partner and I first met, before we were dating, he'd just had eye surgery. I worried about him walking blindly through Portland's streets, so I offered him a ride home one day on the Madsen cargo bike I was borrowing.

I straddled the bike, planted my feet, and clutched the brakes while he clambered into the bucket on the back of the bike. We set off with a wobble, a shake, and a bigger wobble. Within twenty feet, we toppled to the pavement in slow motion. I braced to let the bike down as gently as possible and he rolled almost gracefully onto the pavement. I picked up the bike and we tried again—with the same result.

So I locked up the bike and we walked together instead. Fortunately, getting dumped out of a cargo bike twice wasn't a deal breaker for him. As his vision returned we went on plenty of bike rides together—the most romantic of which invariably involve one of us carrying the other by bike. Here are a few ways this can work:

Side Saddle

Don't have a cargo bike? Don't despair, you can still bring your bike-free date along. There are plenty of ways to double up on a bike, including using the handlebars or top tube as a seat, but the most comfortable and probably safest is the side saddle method. While straddling your bike, plant your feet on the ground, hold tight to your brakes, and ask your date to perch side saddle on your (sturdy) rear rack, feet on the non-drivetrain side. They may want to gently hold onto your waist as you ride, but this can be a stable enough position for casual activities like knitting, reading a book, or waving at gaping bystanders.

Work With the Wobble

Human cargo can be unwieldy and too-heavy, leading to the dreaded wobble that caused me trouble early in my person-carrying days. Practice is key. Ride with heavy loads often enough and you'll used to it. Upper body strength will help you control your bike better in all manner of situations. Take it easy when you brake; as you stop, adjust your pedal position and gearing for an easier start. Finally, communicating with your passenger is key. Let them know when you're getting ready to stop, especially if it'll be a sudden one. Let them know if they're leaning too much or too little into turns.

If you're the passenger on someone's rack or deck, the big thing to remember is to relax, keep centered and steady, and take your pedaler's cues. Don't shift your weight around, and let yourself lean gently with the turns instead of fighting them. Keep your feet out of the wheels and gears. Don't put your feet on the ground, even at stop lights or on turns, unless your pedaler ask you too. When you lift your feet up again, don't push off or try to propel the bike with them—this can seriously throw off the balance.

When I first tipped my date out into the street, I was inexperienced at cargo biking and didn't yet have the instincts or the upper arm strength to keep the bike steady. I've found that any time I carry something particularly heavy or off-balance (like, say, an adult who is a foot taller and 50 pounds heavier than I am), it takes a few blocks for my muscle memory to kick in and compensate for the load. Don't give up too soon—but also, don't be afraid to laugh, admit defeat for the moment, and make another attempt later. Practice really helps.

Trailers

Trailers are less romantic than cargo bikes, but sometimes they really are the best way to carry a passenger, especially if the person is taller and heavier than you, or if they aren't feeling well enough to sit upright and balance themselves. If either you or your passenger is nervous about the ride, seat them on cushions low to the ground rather than up in a chair for better balancing and comfort. If you do use a chair—those fold-up, canvas outdoors chairs with cupholders work great—make sure it's lashed down firmly with taut bungies so it doesn't shift or tip as you ride.

Tandems

A tandem is a bike built for two (or sometimes more) riders, pedaling in unison on a shared drive train. Good communication is paramount for successful tandem riding. One person will be the driver, sitting in front and controlling the steering, pacing, and braking. The other will be the stoker; their job is to navigate, reading maps and calling out directions (and often taking photos), all while providing steady pedaling power. Agreeing on these roles and trusting the other's judgment in their part is key for both parties. So is finding a tandem that can comfortably fit both riders.

Tandem bicycles are renowned as the true test of trust in a relationship. But I wonder how many otherwise perfectly good relationships are damaged by jumping into tandem riding without first actually building up a foundation for that trust by establishing comfortable and mutually agreeable cycling routines and habits together on separate bikes. When that is done, the tandem is transformed from break-up machine to pure romance.

5

FAMILY BICYCLING

"Biking is easy. Having kids is hard!" —Emily Finch, Portland, Oregon, mother of six

My personal experience with family bicycling is nonexistent. But the family bicycle movement is spreading like wildfire, and when I put out a call for advice the response was overwhelming. Much of this chapter consists of the words of the bicycling parents who responded to my request for help.

These folks represent a wide range of experiences, from being the lone cyclists in a rural area to navigating the streets of the bike friendly cities of the Pacific Northwest. Many of them own cars, some only bike recreationally, and others are resolutely car-light or car-free. Some of their advice is complementary, other times they contradict each other. Your own experience will no doubt vary—and there is no right or wrong way to do any of this.

The Family Bicycle Revolution

"We began riding in the summer of 2011 as we transitioned to a car-lite lifestyle. We were hoping to save money on our automobile expenses and live a more community oriented life." —Stacy Bisker, Huntington, West Virginia (kids aged two, five, eight, and nine).

"We ride to spend time together, to take in the sights, smell the ocean, smile at other riders/walkers on the trail. We ride for small adventures to the beach or on the greenbelt trails through the city. We ride for donuts. We ride to piano lessons because it's faster than driving, more scenic, and makes our cheeks rosy." —Kevin Turinsky, Anchorage, Alaska (kid aged twelve and a half)

"Taking the bike is fun! We're all happy and relaxed and talking with the kids doesn't distract me on the bike the way it does in the car. I'm also very motivated by avoiding car traffic and not having to look for and pay for parking. It's also a great form of exercise—and my only form of exercise these days." —Madeleine Carlson, Seattle, Washington (kids aged two and four)

"We try to let our older kids be more free roaming like we were in the 70s. That is definitely not the norm these days for other parents but we usually get kudos, if anything, for that stance. The kids—especially the older ones—almost always prefer to bike." —Dan and Kirsten Kaufman, Portland, Oregon (kids aged four, nine, and twelve)

"Biking is an integral part of our lifestyle, it's faster and more efficient than walking, offers more convenience than relying on bus schedules for most trips and does a great job of keeping us active and in shape. It is easy to sit on the sidelines and bemoan the politics of oil and the injustices of war. I feel that being car-free I am accountable to my children for their future." —Sarah Noga, Arlington, Washington (kids ages one, five, and twelve)

For many of us, riding a bike is sweetly nostalgic of our first taste of freedom and independence. But in recent generations, busy roads and an increasingly indoor, online culture limit kids' range of motion even in their own neighborhoods. In 1969 48 percent of people ages five to fourteen walked or biked to school. By 2009 this number was 13 percent.

Nowadays, when kids come along, even the most resolutely carfree tend to get cars. And it's no wonder. When a baby is born, suddenly at least one parent can't go anywhere without both the kid and a large bag full of diapers, toys, changes of clothes. As kids get older, someone needs to bring them to daycare, school, camp, soccer practice, and birthday parties all over town.

Family bicycles are not yet commonplace in North America, and our streetscapes are often anything but kid friendly.

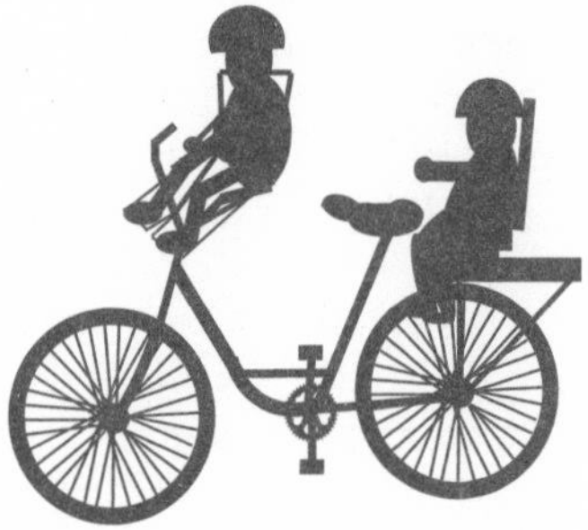

In the face of this adversity, there's a burgeoning family bicycle movement. Many of these bicycling parents determined that their kids grow up with the values, health, and independence that bikes can afford. Others are determined to rediscover their own childhood joy of bicycling and to find a more satisfying, economical, and healthy seat for their daily rounds than the one behind a wheel of a minivan.

Getting Started

"We are new to bicycling and new to family cycling. It was at least ten years ago I was last on a bicycle. We began the process with a lot of thinking, talking, reading, and eventually just trying." —Stacy Bisker, Huntington, West Virginia
"The hardest part about starting was getting over the assumption that it's not possible. [It was always] too far, too steep, too many cars to bike to places we've previously visited by car." —Madeleine Carlson, Seattle, Washington

"The hardest part for me was just good old fashioned fear. The family member well-meaning "what-if" questions kept me up at night. What if the baby gets sick? What if it's snowing? What-if... What about... Well none of that is real. It's just like anything else. If a what-if comes up, we deal with it. The car was no magic-measure of security. If worst case something comes up that makes it impractical to bike or take transit to we can rent a car for a day. Like I said, no big deal." —Sarah Noga, Arlington, Washington

Getting started bicycling with kids, like bicycling on your own, comes with a learning curve—and with an added layer of social and logistical hurdles.

But many parents find that the greatest hurdle is simply deciding to begin. Once they start it quickly becomes hard to remember the obstacles that had seemed insurmountable. In their place, new and unexpected challenges arise, of course. But despite my best efforts to find these out, most parents interviewed for this chapter dwelt far more on the things that became easier and more fun after they began bicycling with their families. I was surprised to hear few complaints about dealing with weather, tantrums, and busy social schedules. In fact, parents expressed that reliance on the bicycle simplified their social life rather than complicating it.

Baby on Board

Pregnancy

Many women continue to ride a bicycle throughout their pregnancy; one woman I know rode her bicycle to the birthing center while in labor, weathering four contractions along her twenty minute ride. The baby came home in a pedicab.

If you have the medical go-ahead to stay physically active during your pregnancy, there is no reason not to continue cycling. Regular physical activity that is built into your day, like bicycling, can help you to handle the physical discomforts that often come with pregnancy, from nausea to swollen feet to mood swings. Cycling can also help you to keep your energy up and maintain your fitness in preparation for birth and what comes after.

As your belly grows, make room for it by switching to a bicycle that allows you a more upright posture, like a cruiser or a Dutch bicycle; or by raising the handlebars on your regular bike. A more upright posture will also help keep you feeling stable as your balance shifts. You may want to add extra gears as well.

Incidentally, the bicycle types that are most comfortable to ride while pregnant are often the ones best suited to carrying children. Shop for family bikes now, before the baby arrives, while you still have the time and energy.

As your pregnancy progresses you'll likely find yourself riding more slowly and avoiding lifting your bike; plan to adjust your routine accordingly. This, too, is good preparation for the pace of life with a baby.

During and after your pregnancy, it's important to listen to your body—and your doctor—when it comes to how much time, if any, you spend on a bicycle.

Riding with Your Infant

You can start riding with your infant right away, unless your pediatrician recommends otherwise. Before your child can hold their head up, their carseat can be carried with you. The car seat can be carried in a number of creative ways. Most parents choose to carry their child either in the bicycle trailer behind them, or in front of them in the bed of a front loader cargo bike. Your car seat carrying solution will depend on what kind of bicycle you plan to ride with your child as they grow.

Bicycle helmets are, in many states, legally required for all children, whenever they are being carried by bicycle. However, they are not manufactured for children under a year old.

But it's best not to combine helmets with carseats—choose one or the other. It is also not safe to put a helmet on a kid who can't hold their head up by themselves. Whatever you do, it is up to you to make the decision about what is best for your family.

Carrying Your Child on Your Bicycle

Want to convert your own bike into a kid carrier by putting a seat on it? There are two basic kinds of child seat: front and rear seats. Many parents of multiple young children have both.

Front Seats

"I highly recommend using a front carrier, where the child sits on the top tube (on a seat that is attached to the top tube, and has a foot rest for them). They are nestled in between your arms so they can't fall off. This allows you talk to them, and gives them a great vantage point to watch everything you are seeing. It allows you to discuss bike riding rules and tips with them in "real time." You can easily talk with them rather than shout over your shoulder like a bike trailer forces you to do." —Kristi Wood, Anchorage, Alaska (mom of a six-year-old)

"I love front seats—it's wonderful to have a small kid right in front. The only change I had to make to my bike to accommodate the seat was a longer stem when my son's knees got too cramped." —Madeleine Carlson, Seattle

Increasingly common, especially for smaller children, are seats that mount on the front of the bike so that a small child can sit between you and the handlebars. These are loved by many parents for the sense of both protection and conversation they afford. They are loved by children for the sheer joy of being at the front of the bike with the world rushing past. (Windscreens can be purchased for some models for rainy or cold days.)

When choosing a front seat, consider how you will mount it to your bike. This depends both on the type of seat and the type of bicycle you plan to use. The basic distinction is that some of these seats mount to your frame—resting on the top tube—while others mount to your steering. The steering-mounted ones can make the bike somewhat more difficult to control, requiring more strength, but some bike frames make them necessary.

Rear Seats

The most widely available seats mount on the rear rack, and can hold kids from a young age up to 75 pounds. These seats come in a lot of varieties; some offer quite a bit of support and may be better for kids that are not yet good at sitting up on their own. Once you've graduated to a rear seat, you can still easily chat with your kid. If you want to keep an eye on them, a handlebar mirror will help.

There are many different kinds of these available. They are typically mounted to your rear rack. You can also mount them to the deck of a longtail cargo bike, though models built for this are limited and most require some fidgeting.

Rear seats are more conventional than front seats as well as easier to find. Your child will eventually grow too large for a front seat, at which point a rear seat may be your best option if they are not yet ready to pedal along with you on a tag-along bike. If you decide to go for a rear seat, consider converting your bike to a longtail (see below). This will improve your overall carrying capacity and give everyone a bit more space.

There are some down sides to rear seats as well. In some cases, a rear seat will interfere with your ability to hang panniers from your rack; others place your child so close to your seat that you will not be able to wear a backpack. Some people find they make the bike top-heavy or hard to balance while getting on and off. And a real downside is that with a child (or even just the seat) on the back of your diamond frame bike, it can be difficult to get on and off. See the section below for tips.

Getting On and Off the Bike

If you ride a diamond frame bike (with a top tube that runs straight between your seat and handlebars), you likely get on and off the bike by swinging your leg over the back tire. Mounting a child's seat on the back of the bike will have the immediate effect of making this simple act immeasurably more difficult. Without too much weight on the bike, you can tip it sideways to lower the bar, but when you have a 30 pound kid on the back this also becomes less of an option.

This is where the brilliance of the step-through frame becomes most apparent. These are highly recommended for anyone who regularly carries kids or cargo on the back of their bicycle.

If you don't have a step-through frame, getting on and off the bike while the kid is on the back may always be awkward. But it can be done.

If your kid is old enough and doesn't need to be strapped in—for instance, if they are sitting on the deck of your longtail—get on the bike first and hold it steady while they climb on.

But most likely, you'll find yourself loading your kid into the child seat and then doing a kind of balancing gymnastics maneuver to thread your leg up and sideways over the top tube while holding the now heavily-loaded bike steady with your arms. Several parents assured me that regular yoga practice really does make this easier.

One way to make getting on the bike easier is to start by standing on a curb while the bike is on the street. For the dismount, Eric Moody of Portland advised, "hold the handle bars and saddle while straddling the bike and then, with great flexibility, pull one knee up and over."

Equipment-wise, just as with any cargo bike, a good, solid kickstand will help a lot with loading and unloading your squirmy cargo, especially if you can kick and un-kick the stand from astride your bike. For even more stability, get a two or three prong model. See chapter four for a more in-depth discussion of these wonderful devices.

Trailers

"When the toddler has fallen asleep, the trailer is a ready made nap bed. I always brought a book in my backpack because it happened quite often. I would get some good reading in and my son would get his afternoon nap." — Travis Wittwer

If you plan to carry your child or children in a trailer, consider purchasing one made specifically for the purpose. These come in narrower models that hold one child, and wider ones that hold two. They feature a canvas seat with a five-point harness (or two) to strap the kids into the bike. Another feature is a rain/sun cover over a high crossbar that provides room for the kid to sit upright. Some trailers are designed to double as strollers, with a removable push bar and third wheel at the front.

All children-specific trailers have two wheels, which makes them stable and extremely difficult to tip over, though speeding down a steep, curvy hill is never recommended with any kind of trailer in tow.

One of the downsides of trailers is they are bulky and not as easy as an unencumbered bicycle to store in say, a cramped garage or bring through the door of a house. Hitching and unhitching a trailer, if you don't bring it with you everywhere, is an extra step that some find annoying on a daily basis. If you live in an area where theft is a concern, trailers are also not always easy to lock up.

See chapter four for more about what to look for in trailers.

Cargo Bikes

A cargo bike combines the best of both worlds. Kids have a bit more room in a trailer, and you can still keep them close, on your own bike, while still being able to carry other kids of cargo, whether it be a diaper bag or groceries.

The basic cargo bike options are described in chapter three. Many more varieties exist; most are wonderful, but not every type is for every person. If you're in the market for one of these bikes, be sure to peruse the section below on cargo bike shopping tips.

Longtails

"We're in the process of outgrowing the city bike so a month ago I got a Surly Big Dummy and love it! It's a lot of bike, but it has a lot of gears. So far the thing I love most is being able to haul two kids and their two balance bikes easily around. Previously, I had to hook up the trailer and shove the balance bikes in there, and I have to admit I hate dragging the trailer around." —Madeleine Carlson, Seattle

"Our typical full family ride uses four bicycles. The two eldest children ride independently, the two youngest ride on our Yuba Mundo with an iBert front seat, PeanutShell rear seat, on the deck, in the trailer, or a combination of any of these. My husband rides his own mountain bike.

When I ride with our four children without another adult the same set up may apply, but recently I have preferred to fit them all on the Yuba Mundo in specific situations. Sometimes the children are exhausted and need to be passengers. Other times the roadways, weather or darkness factors may make riding together a safer option. This is working ok for us right now. It's physically possible thanks to months of riding and gradually adding weight and experimenting with setups." —Stacy Bisker, West Virginia

Longtail bicycles are quickly becoming the classic kid-hauling cargo bikes, proving a sturdy alternative to a minivan. You can read more about them in chapter three; in short, though, a longtail is like a regular bicycle with a frame extension that places the rear wheel several feet farther back and gives the bicycle a lower center of gravity. Most varieties sport a wide deck atop the rear wheelbase, upon which kids can sit, and two large panniers or ledges for carrying hefty items below and alongside the deck.

Longtails are one of the more affordable family bike options. They can be stored in a relatively narrow space and carried up and down stairs if needed. They also ride similarly to regular bikes, though some parents find them difficult to balance when carrying the bulk of the weight above the top deck, as when children are astride.

There are many ways to carry a kid on a longtail. For young children, you can still mount a front seat between you and the handlebars. One or even two rear seats can be mounted to the top deck. The mounting hardware for most rear seats is not compatible with longtails, so some creativity is required to mount the seat securely.

Older children can sit directly on the top deck. They will be most comfortable sitting on a cushion (waterproof ones are designed just for this purpose). It's also a good idea to install footrests and to mount a set of handlebars below your seat for your passenger to hang onto while you ride. A sturdy double kickstand is essential.

If your longtail has a step-through frame, it will make getting on and off much easier. In addition, a bike that affords an upright riding posture will improve your ability to balance the bike comfortably with top-heavy loads.

The best longtails are the Xtracycle and the Yuba Mundo. Yuba makes sturdy, one-piece longtails that can carry many hundreds of pounds. Xtracycle makes a variety of bikes, all longtails, in multiple sizes and for multiple needs. They also make a kit that you can use to convert the bike you already ride into a longtail.

A variation on the longtail is the Madsen bucket bike. This is basically a longtail frame with a large plastic bucket that sits low over the back of the bike and which has seats for as many as four small children. In the bucket, the kids have room to play and can face each other; and being able to carry the weight of the children and cargo lower to the ground improves stability.

Frontloaders

Just as many parents prefer children's seats on the front of their bike rather than the back, many prefer to carry their kids ahead of them in a frontloading cargo bike rather than behind them on a longtail or in a trailer. This positioning facilitates conversation as well as keeping an eye on what your kid is up to and may give you a better shot at preventing them from removing their helmets and throwing their books overboard. Nearly all of the models described below either come with or have available a variety of options for cargo container, locking compartments, seating and straps, and rain/sun covers.

The handling on front-loading bikes often takes some getting used to; the longer the bike the greater the difference with what you are used to. Some parents report that keeping a fully loaded bakfiets upright requires lots of arm strength and feels extremely wobbly and difficult to pedal at first. They quickly become used to the way bakfiets ride, they say, even if it takes a while longer to build the strength to pedal it everywhere. The trick is to steer the bakfiets like a car, rather than leaning it like a bike.

There are several options on the market for front-loading bikes and trikes; most are imported and quite expensive, though these also tend to be the sturdiest and best-designed.

The most well-known front loader in the U.S. is the Dutch bakfiets, with its signature wooden box (note: bakfiets is pronounced "bock-feets" and is the singular form of the noun in Dutch—the plural is bakfietsen). The term literally means "box bike" and is a generic category, but there is also a company by the same name that makes a popular model. Imported bakfietsen have some major advantages: Huge cargo capacity (you can easily carry a reclining adult, or two or more children plus a week of groceries in the box). They are well made, with high-quality, enclosed components, which means that maintenance is rarely needed and you can park them outside in the rain year-round without rust taking over. And they're sturdy, built like tanks.

The major downside to bakfietsen is that they are heavy—as much as 100 pounds empty. They were created for trundling kids and cargo around the pancake-flat Netherlands, and the standard brakes they come equipped with are not suited to stopping at the bottom of a steep hill on a wet day with a full load of cargo. Brakes and gears should be altered to suit your terrain and weather.

The Bullitt, imported from Copenhagen, is another popular front loader option. It's lighter, and it handles more like a conventional bike. It isn't kid-ready out of the box the way a bakfiets is, but it is more flexible in its cargo capacity—it's ready to strap a carseat to or to fit seating (which you must make or buy separately) for a young passenger or two.

Cargo tricycles are another option for front loaders. Tricycles aren't for everyone, but a cargo trike has the advantage of always being upright when you are stopped—no need for a kickstand or to climb on and off at lights. See chapter three for more about cargo trike care and feeding. As for varieties, the Box Bike and Nihola brands, both imported from Europe, are popular and increasingly available. An American made option is the Haley Trike out of Philadelphia; being custom made, these are not necessarily cheaper but are more customizable, allowing for choices in the gearing and box shape.

As family bicycling becomes more popular, there are more and more front loaders on the market that are specifically designed for carrying kids. See the resources page at *EverydayBicycling.com* for more.

Bikes That Your Kids Ride with You

Tag-Alongs

"I was surprised at how quickly they took to it and how much they enjoy it. Their enjoyment of riding is so obvious and so infectious that their two year old brother insists on a turn on the trail-a-bike too when it is out." —Nicole D, DC, nieces aged three and four

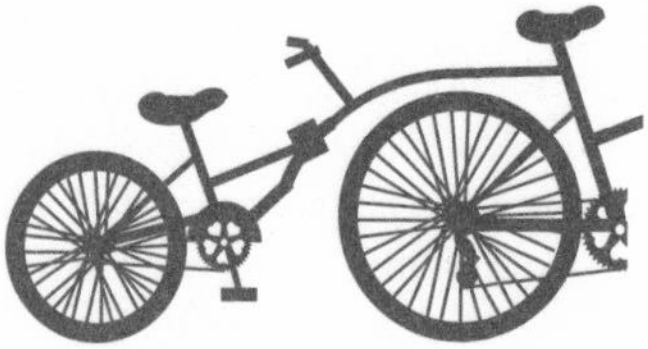

A tag-along is a single wheel, seat, and set of pedals that attaches to the back of your bike. Your child sits on the back and pedals—or doesn't. Like with a tandem, as the young pedaler grows stronger, they can really help power the bike uphill. Tag-alongs are loved by families of young kids who are able to bike on their own, but who can't necessarily go as far or fast as every trip requires. It's also good for kids who get restless sitting passively in a trailer.

When you drop your child off at school via a tag-along, you can remove it from your bike, lock it to a rack, and go about your day unemcumbered. Kids can start on these as soon as they're big enough to ride their own bike; the seats are adjustable so they can keep riding with them up to age eight or even older.

Tag-alongs are widely available used and in good condition. There are several varieties, with different attachments. Most attach to your seat post, which can interfere with your ability to use your rear rack; it can take a few minutes to get used to the feel of riding with one.

Also popular is the Weehoo, which puts your child in a recumbent position-and a seat belt. Another option is the FollowMe, a device that connects your rear wheel with the front of your child's bike, producing the stable ride of a tandem, and freeing up your rear rack,

It is possible to attach some kinds of bicycle trailer to the wheel of a tag-along to increase the capacity (and length!) of your family bike. Look at the weight rating on your tag-along before trying this, and heed it. Tag-along hitches have been known to suddenly fail when asked to exceed their recommended capacity.

Kid Tandems

"Tandems are the most incredible things with kids. We'll set out for a short ride on the tandem, and she'll just sit back there telling me about absolutely everything in her world." —Kevin Turinsky, Anchorage, Alaska

Tandem bikes are especially good for kids who are old enough to ride a bike but for whatever reason are not ready to independently ride their own bicycles everywhere. It's also a frequent and charming sight on longer rides to see parents and teens riding together on a tandem as a bonding activity.

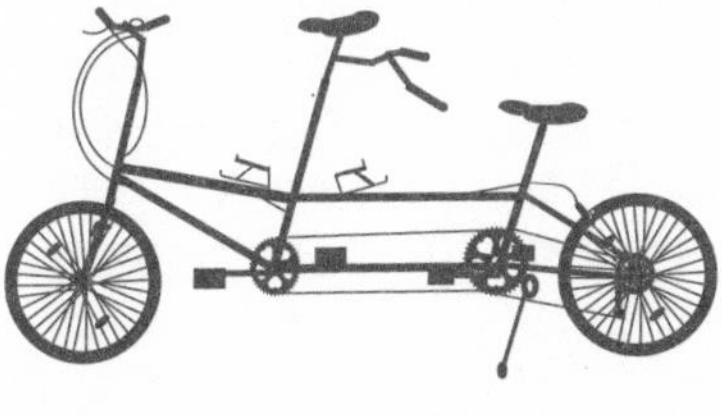

There are a multitude of tandem bicycles out there that are meant to be piloted by an adult joined by either one or even two children. These bikes are not cheap, but they can be adjusted for growing kids and can be used for years.

In most of these the adult rides in the front, piloting the bike, while one or two children ride behind, stoking.

Newer types of family tandem allow the kid to ride in the front while the adult behind them maintains control over steering and braking. These bikes often are shorter than tandems (meaning the pilot in the rear can see around corners better than you might think) and at times resemble a hybrid between a tandem and a bike with a child's seat in the front, and a front loader where the passenger can pedal.

Kid tandems are typically designed so that the kid does not have to be pedaling for the bicycle to go forward—the adult can be doing all the work. Because these are similar to regular bicycles you can still put a rack and panniers over the front and rear wheels. Some parents will add on even more kids by putting a child seat over the rear wheel, or between them and the handlebars, or by towing a trailer or a tag-along behind.

A Note on Electric Assists

Electric assists can be fitted to many cargo bike set-ups, and some specialty cargo bicycle shops also offer excellent electric assist options. Chapter three includes more details about the pros and cons of the electric assist. When it comes to family bicycling, some parents find an extra boost going up the hills they traverse regularly makes all the difference; others find the unit's battery to be heavy and bulky, and one extra thing to keep track of.

Shopping for Family Bikes

"For us, having the opportunity to test ride bicycles with the conditions we encounter daily would have been the greatest benefit. My five-minute test ride on the Yuba in Columbus, Ohio without my family is nothing like what we deal with adding moving weight and hills. When we were selecting a bicycle, we reached out to other bicycling families around the country and we are most happy we did. No one here had the information or the bicycles. It's been a lonely adventure in that respect, but one that has give us perspective and passion." —Stacy Bisker, Huntington, West Virginia

Family bicycling is still relatively new to North America, which means that family bikes and gear can be expensive. Bikes and seats often need to be imported; locally made varieties tend to be manufactured in small quantities; either way the prices can seem sky-high.

Keep in mind that when it comes to cargo bikes you get what you pay for. If you're on a tight budget, look for a used bargain before you settle for a cheap knockoff. The good news is that the same factors that lead to high prices also mean that most cargo bikes on the market right now are so well made that even heavily used ones will often still be in great condition to meet your family's needs for many more years.

Buying a new cargo bike can be the equivalent of investing in a used car, in both utility and price. But unlike a car, a utility bike needs to not just fit your passengers and stuff—it needs to fit you comfortably, as well as any other adults who will be piloting the bike. It also needs to have suitable gearing and brakes for the type of terrain you'll be riding on.

Test riding a bike before you purchase it is essential, especially if it is a pricey investment that you plan to use as a major family vehicle. That said, many families just read up about their options and jump in, and things work out well. Cargo bikes hold their value, and if your first attempt doesn't work out, another family will likely be very happy to take it off your hands.

If you live in a city that boasts a specialty cargo bike shop, then you're in luck. These shops tend to have small selections tended by knowledgeable and helpful owners. An increasing number of regular local bike shops carry one or more lines of cargo and kid-specific bikes. Ask at yours to see if they have anything for you to try. If not, you may need to get creative.

Another option is to find other early adopters near you who are willing to let you try their bikes out. If nobody in your town rides a bakfiets, maybe a family an hour away has one. The Internet is a great resource for finding bicycling families.

Another option is to go to where the bikes are. If you have a vacation or business travel planned to a city where there are bike shops that carry cargo bikes, then plan to test ride as many as you can during that time, preferably with your kids and something equivalent to a couple of bags of groceries on board. Some families plan their vacations specifically around this goal.

Maintaining Your Family Bike

While you seek out the bike setup of your dreams, conduct a simultaneous search for the mechanic of your dreams. The good news is that the more expensive the bike, the less maintenance it is likely to need. European imports are built to last forever with minimal care. The drivetrain is internal, the tires are as durable and puncture-proof as bike tires can be, and even the chain is enclosed in a case. This is a good thing, because they are extra difficult to work on and often require specially imported parts and tools.

Even if you don't need to take your bike in every month for a flat tire or squeaky brake, you will still need to do a tune-up once a year to keep the wheels spinning smoothly and the brakes stopping you safely. So unless you have a motivated handy person under your own roof, it's a good idea to start feeling out your local bike shops and seeing if one of them has a mechanic eager to take on the challenge of caring for your new ride.

Teaching Your Kids to Ride Independently

Balance Bikes

Probably the best way—and definitely the cutest—to start your kid off learning to bicycle when they are tiny is with a balance bike, also called a scoot bike or a run bike. These resemble most of all the velocipedes of two hundred years ago—they have two wheels, handlebars and a seat, but no gears or pedals. The kid sits on the seat and propels themself forward with a running motion, also using their feet to stop. You walk or ride along with them, teaching them the fine art of stopping at intersections, looking for cars, and riding with others.

Learning to ride a balance bike tends to be the best way to prepare a child for the transition to a pedal bike. True to their name, they teach the most difficult part of bicycling—balance—in a way that tricycles and training wheels don't.

If you have an older child who is learning to ride, or if you don't want to invest in a balance bike that will be quickly outgrown, you can get similar results, though with somewhat more ankle-bruising potential, by removing the pedals from the regular two wheeler your child will eventually ride. Once they are comfortable

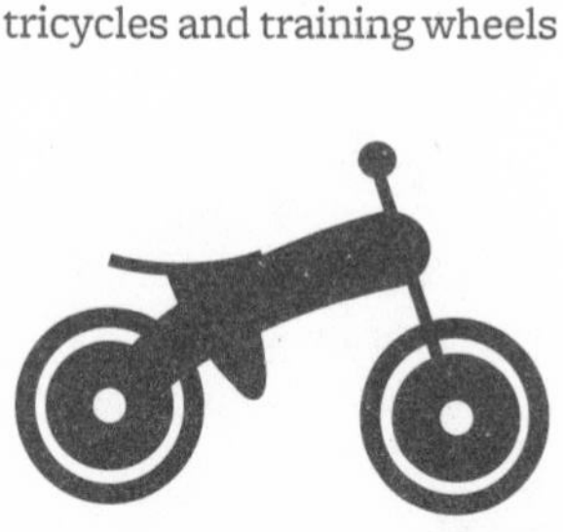

scooting and gliding around this way, put the pedals back on and they'll get the hang of it in no time.

Training Wheels

Training wheels are still the standard way to start your kid out riding a bike. Here is how training wheels work: You install them on a two-wheeler so that they hover an inch off the ground when the bike is upright. The idea is that if the kid tips one way or the other, for instance while turning, the training wheel on that side can carry them for a minute until they are able to balance themselves upright again. Raise the wheels incrementally as the new bicyclist gains skills and confidence, until eventually they are no longer needed.

Training wheels are not an ideal solution for everyone. The most timid new cyclists tend to treat a bike mounted with training wheels as a tricycle, riding on three points—this does not help them learn balance or confidence and makes for an uncomfortable ride. If you are not having good luck with training wheels or would like to bypass them altogether, then for younger kids go with a balance bike, and for older kids and teens see the first chapter for tips on learning to ride.

The Big Kid Bike

"I think the key is understanding the child, knowing when you need to go exactly at their pace and when it is ok to push just a little bit further. Kids like to say 'I can't' a lot. I have learned to ignore that and say 'but see, you just did' a lot. It is amazing how far a little encouragement goes." —Nicole Donnelly, Washington, DC

How old do you have to be to learn to ride? The answer varies, sometimes wildly—every kid learns at their own pace. Some are ready to roll as soon as they can toddle, while others aren't comfortable getting on a bike until they are in their teens or older.

You'll likely know when your own kids are ready. When that happens, how do you teach them to ride safely and confidently?

Teaching Your Kid to Ride

Doug Smart teaches bike safety to school kids in Corvallis, Oregon. Here are his guidelines:

• Model expected behavior. Kids aren't interested in things like formative vs. mature brains—if you expect them to wear their helmets, then you need to wear yours.

• Consistency. All the safety checks and behaviors need to be done the same way every time so they can become lifelong habits.

• Responsibility. For many kids bicycling is one of their first opportunities to interact with adults on a nearly equal basis. They are responsible for their own choices and the consequences of those choices to themselves and others.

• Get comfortable! If you're a nervous role model, your kids will learn to be nervous when they ride. This may mean doing family rides on off-street paths for a while as you both build skills.

• Trust your kids. Emphasize safety and offer some coaching and then shut up for a bit. Give them space to make mistakes.

• Consider asking for help. It is not abdicating parental responsibility to ask a friend to help out or to put your kids into a class to learn bike skills. Often kids will listen better to an adult who isn't their parent. Just make sure you and that other adult are reinforcing each other.

Riding Together

Riding with your kid, especially when they're just starting out, will present a learning curve for you as well as for them.

Start with short rides, stopping while it's still fun, before your kid is tired or overwhelmed. Teach one or two new ideas at a time.

What you do is even more important than what you say. When riding with your kid, whether on separate bikes, or with them on the back of your bike, it's important to be confident and consistent. See chapter one for basic skills and safety practices. If it is your habit to stop when it's necessary, signal your turns, hold your line, and know how to safely handle difficult traffic situations, then your kid will learn to ride safely without much instruction. Conversely, if you're a timid or aggressive rider, or if you treat stop signs differently when you're riding on your own, your kid will pick up on that and ride that way as well.

One question some parents have is where to ride in relation to their child. As with everything else, there's no right answer. Ride in front to control the pace, show the way, and ensure that the kid is going to stop. Ride behind to keep an eye on your kid, and protect their wiggle zone. If you say "stop" and the kid doesn't stop, you can zoom up ahead of them.

Choosing Kids' Bikes

"Nothing too complicated. Balance bikes are great for really small kids. Getting into grade school a standard bike with the pedals temporarily removed will serve the same purpose. A multi-speed bike is ok if they don't worry about shifting until they have the basics down. Beyond that, it needs to be something that can be easily adjusted to fit." —Doug Smart, Corvallis, Oregon

"If you're going to build your kid a bike, make one they'll want to be seen on." —Kevin Turinsky, Anchorage, Alaska

Every year it gets a little easier to find new bikes for kids. Go to a bike shop you trust and look for everything you would want on your own bike to make it comfortable for the type of riding your kid will be doing. Make sure it fits comfortably, and add fenders if your kid will be riding in wet weather, and a rack or basket for carrying things. You'll also want to get them a helmet and a lock for the bike, and if they'll ever be riding at night they'll need lights. A bell is even more fun and satisfying for kids than for adults.

There is a glut of cheaply assembled bicycles available at big box stores—these are tempting, especially when kids are growing quickly. But they are not designed to be ridden farther than the end of your driveway and even at such close range they tend to fall apart quickly. Buying a kids' bike from a local bike shop will help ensure a higher level of both quality and service as your child begins their independent bicycling life.

Another good option is to go vintage. Most bikes used to be built to last. Your chances of finding an old banana seat cruiser in good condition will go up considerably the less popular bicycling is where you live. You'll need to get any vintage bike thoroughly tuned up and you may need to replace all the rubber before it's road ready, but this can be an attractive and relatively affordable option.

Used bikes of a more recent era are also often a good option. If your kid doesn't have an older sibling to inherit an outgrown bicycle from, perhaps a friend or neighbor is ready to move on. Also, community bike projects or co-ops often have a surplus of kid's bikes available to build up.

Kids grow, and it's safe to assume that most kids' bikes won't be with you for long, which is another reason to invest in a good quality one that you'll be able to resell.

But make sure that the bicycle you invest in doesn't have too much room to grow. Trying to balance on a bike is tricky enough, and it's even harder when you have trouble reaching the pedals, much less the ground.

A final option for kids once they get into grade school is folding bikes. The seatpost and reach are fairly adjustable, though length tends to be a bit more of an issue. If a kid is reaching too far, they'll have trouble controlling the bicycle. But once your child is able to comfortably ride a folding bicycle, they'll be able to keep the same bike through adulthood.

Family Biking Logistics

Safety

Safety is a relative concept, and deeply disputed. It's hard to shake the idea that cars are safe, armored vehicles and this feeling of safety has led to something of an arms race in the size and weight of family vehicles. But statistically speaking, children are in more imminent physical danger while in and around motor vehicles than in any other situation. The lasting effects of inactivity and social isolation are even greater in children than in adults.

In reality, we each have a different threshold when it comes to what feels safe and what doesn't. And whatever your theories about safety, the reality of the roads on which you travel will likely have an even greater impact on your decisions about bicycling. Here are just a few perspectives:

"We have found most every town can be traversed by bicycle. It is a matter of knowing where to go, being flexible, having an understanding of your community and its life pattern. We are familiar with which streets have more car traffic, where to go at night for better lighting, less pot holes or where the side walk may be the favorable and safer location. All of this has taken time and practice. There are places we would not travel by bicycle with our children, but would go there alone or with other adults. Our children can be more unpredictable on a bicycle and some roads require a lot more attention. Some places are too far for their endurance. Sometimes we travel late at night

and we prefer to know we can get everyone home without them falling asleep at the handle bar." —Stacy Bisker, West Virginia

"I think safety has to come first when you are taking a child with you, and that can be an absolute deal breaker. We lived in central Texas until Cora was one year old, and cycling with her was completely out of the question. The issue was cultural as much as it was about infrastructure. This was one of many factors in our decision to relocate to a place like Portland. It's completely different here. Getting started was so easy. Now the challenge is choosing to get out there in the rain and dark whenever we can with her. Honestly, the car is always there as a backup" —Chris Trahey, Portland (kid aged two and a half)

"It took Tyler a little while to get used to wearing a helmet, but we made it clear it was necessary and now he doesn't even think twice about wearing it." —Kristi Wood, Anchorage, Alaska (kid aged six)

"We have to assume that we are completely invisible and most of the time it seems like we are." —Sarah Noga, Arlington, Washington

"Have the belief that kids will be safe and that a parent has the skill to keep them safe. Routes should be planned; riding in traffic should be taught and practiced; and riding on a street involves a level of focus that is different than riding on a sidewalk." —Travis Wittwer, Portland

Weather

"Many parents seem to think children are fragile humans that must be sheltered from the elements, when in our opinion, as long as you dress your child appropriately, there is no reason to shield them from inclement weather. We think it's good for kids to learn how to be comfortable and enjoy themselves in 'bad' weather." —Kristi Wood, Alaska

"We don't go out with children in heavy rain. We go out in light to moderate rain when we must, and we go out prepared. Clothing has certainly been something we have been investing in. All the children now have waterproof

jackets. We haven't bothered with waterproof pants yet, but use snow pants in colder weather." —Stacy Bisker, West Virginia

A number of parents have confided to me that Portland's incessant rain seems to bother them far more than it bugs their kids; several said their kids actually love to ride on the back of the bike in the rain.

The same weather advice given for adult riders in chapter two applies to young ones. Drink a lot of water and play it safe in very hot weather; in cold or rainy weather, focus primarily on staying warm rather than staying dry.

Fenders are a must when you have kids on your bike in wet weather, or in a trailer or tagalong behind you. Rain and/or sun covers can be purchased for many cargo bikes, and are well worth the extra investment. Bring a towel to wipe off bike seats that have gotten wet while the bike is parked. Kids who are sitting still on a bike will get colder than ones pedaling, and need warmer clothes; but impermeable rain gear is less likely to be a problem. Waterproof ponchos with hoods are good raincoats for growing kids, and can be draped over the bike seat along with the kid to keep water from pooling below them; a drawstring sewn into the bottom hem can prevent it from blowing around.

Keeping Kids Happy on the Bike

"It's okay to bribe them with treats. Then they sit on the bike and eat cookies instead of trying to take off their helmets." —Emily Finch, Portland, Oregon

"Having a word game makes it easy so that there is no time to complain. We would play word games like do the alphabet with bike related parts or items we see around us. My sons' favorite was each of us in turn taking turns adding to a story. Snacks also make it easy. It is hard to complain about being on a bike when dad has crackers, a bar, or apple slices." —Travis Wittwer, Portland, Oregon

"The occasional trip in the car or on the bus is all it takes for me to appreciate how much easier the bike is. The two kids tend to argue in the car, but the moment we're on the bike, everything is joyful. We notice more exciting things—exciting to toddlers and preschoolers, that is—boats, train tracks, cement mixer trucks, etc." —Madeleine Carlson, Seattle, Washington

Always having snacks and water on hand for both you and the kids on your bike will significantly improve everyone's experience. Bringing toys and books along can also help keep your kid occupied in the trailer or bucket. If your child is a thrower, tie their toy or sippie cup down—try one of those spiral lanyards. Make sure the tie-down isn't long enough to get caught in a wheel if the item is chucked overboard.

Life Logistics and Scheduling

"The flattest route is always better than the shortest route." —Emily Finch, Portland

"We have to plan out grocery stops better and do less of the 'I forgot one thing let me drive back to the store and get it' kind of impulsive trips. Uh, yeah...we get to eat a lot more, too." —Sarah Noga, Arlington, Washington

"One trick is to encourage play dates that are close to our house, so that we have less distance to go." —Kristi Wood, Anchorage

"I need to get over my tendency to apologize for having to schedule around the extra time it sometimes takes to arrive by bike." —Madeleine Carlson, Seattle
"We have tried hard to not replace many of our former auto destinations, enjoyments, or habits but found that we do end up declining some party invitations because of distance, or not running out for plumbing parts seventeen miles away. We have learned to prioritize our time and energy, something we had often been on the track to do, but increased our conscientious efforts with this transition. We may drive to a far away party, but it is because the host is a good friend, not just because we received a classmate invitation. We once waited three days for the local hardware store to open and made do with just one working toilet. In either situation, there were only benefits to be found." —Stacy Bisker, West Virginia

The pace of life changes by bicycle; and this becomes even more true once you have kids. Getting kids out the door no matter what vehicle you use can be a challenge; by bicycle it can become more time consuming, as extra things like rain gear and helmets need to be found and adjusted. Bicycling outside of the neighborhood also tends to take longer when you're carrying kids.

Logistical issues result in many bicycling families simply going fewer places and partaking in fewer extracurricular activities. For many parents and their kids, this is a net positive, resulting in less time on the go and more time to play.

Bicycling families often—though by no means always—include one parent who works from home or part time, or whose full time job is child rearing. This arrangement is frequently made financially feasible by the choice to sell a car or drive it less.

Creating Community

"If there are local biking groups, go on a group ride. Kidical Mass rides are wonderful to ride with...or just meet them at their end point if you're not ready to climb aboard your bike just yet. But many cities have group rides that aren't specifically family-oriented, but are geared towards new riders or riders of all abilities. Seeing real people out there is great, but it's also inspiring to connect with other biking parents online: read blogs, tweets, join Facebook groups, whatever it takes to see that people out there are getting out there every day—and we'd love to have you join us!" —Madeleine Carlson, Seattle

"Find opportunities wherever you are, as close to home as possible, and just start riding. If you feel that the community or infrastructure is a roadblock to safe and fun cycling, consider what it says about the community and then do one of two things: become the champion of change or relocate." —Chris Trahey, Portland

"If you're not already, get active in every aspect of transportation and development planning in your community that you can. The earlier the better. This will allow you to have a positive and beneficial impact on your transportation choices and options, as well as allow your children to see how the process works and how to improve it." —Kevin Turinsky, Anchorage, Alaska

"Joining a local Kidical Mass ride or creating your own weekend ride with other interested families is a great way to both create community as well as learn from each other". —Travis Wittwer, Portland

Meeting other bicycling families often leads to opportunities to socialize at your own pedal-powered pace, as well as to share information, resources, and to get involved in improving bicycling conditions in your community. There are any number of ways to connect with other families; two of the most successful in recent years have been Kidical Mass and the developement of the concept of bike trains.

Kidical Mass has sprung up in the last several years and happens in cities all over the country. It's a short, slow-paced ride, in which families with kids of all ages and skills, on all kinds of bikes, ride together in the street. Usually these rides are short, stick to relatively low-traffic streets, and involve a park on one end and an ice cream shop on the other. Anybody can organize a Kidical Mass ride—see tips in chapter six. Like its namesake, Critical Mass, it's a lot of fun as well as being a valuable venue to meet other families and start to get comfortable riding in the street.

"Bike trains/bike buses are useful. When I took the kids to school via bike, we went about half of the time with a bike bus. It made our numbers larger so we were a better presence on the road and provided a sense of community; connecting my sons with other capable adults." —Travis Wittwer, Portland

Bike trains and walking school buses aren't a new idea, but they're enjoying a surge in popularity as a way for kids to walk and bike to school with adult supervision and safety in numbers. Sometimes they're organized by local college students, other times parents or school volunteers take turns leading as many as a hundred kids by bike through neighborhood streets to school. They tend to meet at a park and make their way to school through back streets, sometimes stopping to pick up more kids along the way. A good number of adults are on hand to help out wobbly riders, ensure safety, and cheer on the young participants.

More Tips

A single chapter can hardly encapsulate all there is to say about family bicycling. The topic demands its own book—until that can be written, I'll leave you with these wise words of advice from our pioneering experts.

"Eighty percent of bike commuting is above the shoulders. It's developing the mind-set that overcomes all the little excuses that tend to keep us from doing new things." —Kristi Wood, Anchorage

"We get lots of questions and inquiries on just about every trip. I feel this is my opportunity to demystify our car-free lifestyle." —Sarah Noga, Arlington, Washington

"Kickstands get treated as an 'accessory' but with family bikes, they really ought to be standard, and sturdy, and ideally, two-footed. Kids will climb around on bikes." —Katie Proctor, Portland (kids aged one and three)

"Bells. Kids love a good bell and the giving of a bell can be a token of accomplishment—you have done great and are ready for having a bell for when we ride in the street. And correctly adjusted helmets. Low on the forehead." —Travis Wittwer, Portland

"Make it special. My nieces and I have matching bike bracelets and matching bike tee shirts and we call ourselves a girl bike gang. Boys can ride with us, but they can't join! We don't always wear them, but it is something we have that creates more of a bond." —Nicole Donnelly, Washington, DC

"Families with special needs can do this too!" —Kath Youell, Portland, Oregon (kids aged five and seven)

"Start young and tell your kids why you prefer cycling. Get the right gear and consider moving to a neighborhood that is conducive to walking and cycling. The rent may be higher but it will save you money in the long run, increase your quality of life, and lower your worry factor." —Dan and Kirsten Kaufman

"Just start slow and get out there!" —Madeleine Carlson

6

GET ORGANIZED!

The first bike event I organized was terrifying. It was a cold November night and I was absolutely certain both that nobody would show up and that a large crowd would be there looking to me for direction. I put off leaving minute by minute, unnecessarily re-reading the organizing and publicity emails, counting the homemade signs rolled in a tube in my bike basket, wondering if the nausea I suddenly felt was a good enough excuse to stay in.

But finally I forced myself to go, rolling up to the meeting point ten minutes late. My second-greatest fear had come true—there was a sizeable crowd, two reporters with notebooks, and a film crew in an SUV, all looking at me and waiting for direction. Within minutes, I had made several new friends, given my first television interview, and was on my bike, happily doing the thing I love most—riding through Portland's streets with a crew of chatting, cheery fellow riders.

The goal wasn't the same for everyone there. Some wanted to raise awareness about inconsistent police enforcement of bicycle laws. Others wanted to send a message to cyclists to stop at every stop sign, and yet others wanted to send the same message to car drivers. For many of us, getting together to ride, meeting other riders, and talking about cycling was the underlying objective. We didn't have to agree on the issue at hand in order to want to make sure the public conversation about bicycling reflected the complexities that we encountered every day on the road.

Bikes and Community

Bicycling can be empowering and transformative on a purely personal level. But it can also get a bit lonely, especially if you live somewhere it hasn't caught on yet. When you're out there alone, indignities tend to pile on: hostile drivers, misinformed police officers, unsafe streets and dangerous road crossings. Some people handle these difficulties by moving—across town, or perhaps even to a new city or country. Many others stay right where they are and work to improve bicycling conditions—much to the benefit of many a place that ten years ago would not have been seen as a likely bike-friendly community.

Many riders quickly discover the value of riding with others. Having a friend, coworker, or spouse to ride with, or even just to talk with about riding, is one of the primary factors that helps people start riding and keep it up. Having several friends, or a community, is what turns cycling into a way of life and allows it to become a widespread movement.

Subcultures are constantly emerging around bikes. You're probably already familiar with the sight of lycra'd out recreational riders pedaling around back country roads on a sunny weekend. Then there are the lawyers who go on hard and fast competitive lunchtime rides. Messengers seek glory in urban alleycat races. Grassroots bike festivals bring people together in cities around the world for purposes as wide-ranging as bike commuter breakfasts, educational sightseeing tours, and political protests. Critical Mass, though controversial, has served an essential function as an incubator for many bicycle organizations and events with more mainstream appeal. Cultures rise up around bike polo, welding and riding tall bikes, bicycle dance, riding restored vintage bikes, bicycle-themed art, teen bike programs, and anything else you can imagine.

Riding in a group allows you to check out what kind of bikes other people are riding, what they wear when they ride, what routes they take, how they handle turns and stops and hills, and to compare notes and share resources.

Even if you're the only person you know who rides a bike, the Internet can be a huge boon in the same way. There are many online forums where the smallest topics in cycling are discussed and argued about to an absurd—and extremely helpful—level of detail.

The value of building a bicycle community is substantial on several levels. Being around other riders—on the roads, in the office, at the bar or coffeeshop, or online—is validation. Especially if you're a pioneer, as a transportation cyclist, or riding with kids, or riding at all, you will benefit greatly from regular reminders that you aren't the only one, that your choice to ride is sane and relatively safe one, that you aren't blocking traffic, and that someday in the not-so-distant future you might have a lot of two-wheeled company.

Getting Organized

Beginning to ride a bike has been the occasion for many an ordinary citizen to become a dedicated attendee of city council meetings, documenter of road conditions, and amateur urban planning expert. The effects of these efforts are palpable, and usually of great benefit to the surrounding community, bike riders and otherwise. As you learn, don't forget to talk—and listen—to others. You can do a lot on your own, but your advocacy will have a more lasting impact when it clearly comes from the community.

Starting a Group

Maybe you want to do more than just go on one bike ride. Maybe you'd like to start a group that meets regularly and can discuss issues online as well. Forming a group is a powerful tool for tapping into the energy in your community for improving bicycling conditions, or just to meet other people who ride bikes.

The Old Fashioned Way

It used to be that if you wanted to get a group of people together who share a passion for the same issue or cause, you would reach them by leaving fliers at places they were likely to spend time.

Even in the age of the Internet, this method still works—and sometimes works even better than a social media campaign. If you want to hold a meeting to talk about a local intersection that's dangerous for cycling or to start a social riding group, it's easy to create and photocopy an invitation and post it in bike shops, coffee shops, offices, student unions, on bike parking racks, and anywhere else where a rider or potentially interested person might see them.

Then show up at the appointed time and place prepared with paper and pens so you can take notes and gather everyone's contact information.

If only one other person shows up, you've got the seeds of something real. If you get three or more attendees, you have a movement.

If you are holding a meeting about a particular issue and are concerned that someone will come who opposes your effort and wants to derail it, make sure you have your allies and arguments lined up ahead of time. But don't forget to listen to your project's opponents; their concerns are likely valid, and your efforts will be all the stronger if you can find a way to work together.

Blogs

Have a way with words, or with computers? Are you inclined to observe, listen, and report? There's a real niche out there for bicycle blogging. The most successful blogs are either hyper-local, reporting on the details of roads, issues, events, and people in a particular region, city, or even neighborhood. Other bloggers choose a topical niche, such as vintage bicycles, biking with children, or analyzing legal issues in bicycling, and are able to find an audience and make their mark in that way.

Setting up a website is easy, and can be as simple as signing up for a free site through Blogger or Wordpress. Gaining an audience requires more work and requires regularly producing topical, readable content, reaching out to potential readers and to other writers and businesses that serve them, and finding a rhythm that doesn't burn out you, the blogger.

Established bloggers often are able to increase the amount of time they dedicate to the blogs by monetizing them. The bike bloggers most successful at earning a living from their work tend to be ones who have created an essential community resource that provides readers with opportunities to connect with each other and tap into broader happenings in the blogger's chosen realm.

Forums and Email Lists

Plain old email lists, where you hit "reply-all" can get unwieldy quickly once you have more than three or four people involved. Email groups and lists, meetup groups, or listservs, are the next step up; they're centrally organized, people can choose to add and remove themselves, and a moderator can ensure that things run smoothly and spam doesn't take over.

Forums are similar, but instead of every message being delivered to every member's inbox, participants must actively go to the forum's page and look at what others' have posted. Forums are excellent when more people are involved and working on diverse projects or discussing diverse interests that don't necessarily overlap.

Both forums and listservs are excellent when there's a community of people in a similar area or with a niche interest who want to have regular interactions or ongoing conversation. These are great organizing tools for channeling many peoples' energy into a project or into discussing issues. People can share their research, ideas, and information spontaneously. They can also propose and begin organizing rides and events, or toss around proposals and ideas to keep each other inspired/encouraged/motivated. These are especially great when their members can also get together in person regularly, though it doesn't have to be that way.

Meetings

If at all possible, it's always better to get people together in person, even if not frequently, on a regular basis. Whether you are planning an event, brainstorming a lobbying session, founding a new organization or just having a social event over beer/hot chocolate, meeting up in person is important. This is where having a listserve, server, or blog comes in handy because it can get people together and then allow people who were unable to meet to see all of the info discussed in the event displayed in one place.

Meetings are where the best schemes happen. Make sure everyone has a chance to introduce themselves. Make them fun. Go for a ride afterwards.

Unless your meetings are merely social, don't have them without a specific, clear goal in sight. It helps to have a facilitator *and* a note-taker who can then put notes online or otherwise share them with the group.

How to Lead a Ride

Leading a bike ride can be done for fun, to meet people, for a political purpose, or just to ride. Everyone on the ride doesn't need to share the same motivation. A ride can be a great way to get people together, build community, and get a different feeling for the streets of your community. You can safely ride on streets you would not necessarily brave on your own.

Step one: Choose a theme or a purpose for your ride. Are you riding to a destination, like a coffee shop, bar, a movie or to testify at city hall? Or is the purpose of your ride to explore nearby trails, learn about local history, or see bike infrastructure? You could also have a ride for a social reason—like to get together with other people who have cargo bikes, host a singles ride, or just for fun among friends.

Step two: Chose a date and time for the ride. Make sure it doesn't conflict with the date and time of another event your riders may be interested in joining. If it does, see if you can start/end at the same location. Also choose a starting location. If it's a business or public gathering place, call ahead to make sure they'll open and as a courtesy to let them know there might be a rush.

Step three: Plan your route. Ride your route in advance. Tailor the route (such as which streets it goes down) depending on your participants. Is it an "in your face" ride to go down main streets to make a statement, or is it a social ride for little kids to get ice-cream and ding their bells? Scout out your route again a day or two before the actual ride to make sure there is no construction or other obstacles have popped up. It's good to know what turns/intersections you'll go through and whether or not you'll need ride helpers. Sometimes it's nice and safer to have people block intersections on larger rides.

Step four: Promote your ride. Make a flier, promote it on the internet, send it out over email lists, tell your friends, ask organizations to spread the word, or you could even send out a press release. It's an obvious thing to say, but people often forget to mention vital information on posters and in emails. Make sure you include: name, date, starting time, starting place, ending place, phone number and any other information people need to know (like who is the ride appropriate for?).

If you want your ride to show up in newspapers and community calendars, you may need to let them know a month in advance. For T.V., radio, and blogs, let reporters know at least a week in advance and give them a reminder the day before. Of course if you are not planning your ride to be very big, you may not need to do all of this, but even if you want just ten people to come, you'll need to make sure they have all of the information.

Step five: The ride itself. Arrive at the meeting place early. It'll be your job to make sure the ride leaves more or less on time. You may want to leave five to ten minutes after the announced start time to allow stragglers to join you, but any longer than that and people get restless. For a ride of more than a dozen or so people, it's a good idea to have one person leading the pack and at least one other person who knows the route who can bring up the rear in case someone gets a flat tire or is otherwise going slowly. If the group gets split up by red lights or flat tires, make sure the people at the front know that is happening, so they can wait for everyone else. Unless it's a race, keep it slow! There's a big difference between recreational rides for fitness and social rides for exploration, chatting, or protest.

Step six: After the ride, thank everyone for coming. If there's a good feeling and people want to keep hanging out, head to a bar or coffee shop. Start planning the next step!

Step seven: Follow up. Set a date for any follow-up activities, the next ride, or meeting and let participants know about it. Add new folks to the email list or let them know where they can find more information, and make sure they have a way to contact each other. If any members of the media covered your event, be sure to thank them.

Advocacy

If you are inclined to love diplomatic endeavors and untangling complex and contradictory technical issues, you might be a born advocate.

If you have a local bicycle or active transportation advocacy organization, contact them to find out how to get involved. Most offer basic volunteer opportunities like stuffing envelopes, or staffing the registration table at fundraising rides. These are great ways to get to know an organization, see how and if you might fit in to higher level volunteer positions, or see opportunities for new advocacy that their organization does not address. Depending on your skills and interests, you might end up helping organize events, monitoring legislative hearings, drafting position papers, or sitting on a committee dedicated to fundraising, outreach, or strategic planning.

If there is no local organization whose work appeals to you, consider starting one. Even if you are not so inclined, you can still be an effective advocate on your own by testifying at your local city hall, writing a letter to the editor, lobbying your state (or national) representatives, getting signatures for voter referendums, or even running for office yourself.

Approaching City Hall

Sometimes city hall is ready to help you; the powers that be just may not realize there is a need. In other cases, there may be obstructions. Your approach will depend on your local political climate, who is responsible for creating safer conditions for bicycling, and how receptive they are to actually doing so.

Sometimes advocacy can be as simple as a phone call. If there is a major pothole on your bike route, glass in the bike lane on a major street, or an intersection along your route where people in cars routinely run the red light, you can call and report it; look online or in the blue pages for the proper number. If your request is fulfilled, be sure to write a thank you note.

Sometimes a simple phone call or letter is all you need to encourage major projects as well, like a bike lane on a major road or a crosswalk in front of a school.

If you have a more complicated project, or if repeated requests haven't been effective, it's time to get organized.

Your first step is to decide what to ask for. Perhaps it's a bike lane on a busy road that is about to be repaved—this is an excellent time to make infrastructure changes because the cost of re-striping the road already needs to be spent. Other potential asks include lowering the speed limit on a street near a school, having bike parking installed in front of the library, hosting a ciclovia-style open streets event, or dedicating a certain percentage of the transportation budget to bicycling infrastructure.

Your next step is to do the research and talk to the stakeholders. Familiarize yourself with local laws. Perhaps your city has a transportation plan or even a bicycle master plan. Try to meet with the mayor or the person on the city council in charge of transportation, with the city-employed transportation planner in charge of bicycling infrastructure (if there is one), and with any business owners, residents, or other people who might be affected or have a direct interest in this project.

This is not the time to make demands, but rather to build relationships. From these conversations, you will gain helpful contacts and get a sense of who will be an ally and in what capacity. You may also find that you need to change what you are asking for. For instance, maybe there isn't room for a bike rack in front of the library, but the owners of the pharmacy next door have the extra sidewalk width and wouldn't be opposed to a rack so long as they don't have the responsibility of maintaining it.

Your next step is to decide how to go forward. Often, your meeting with the mayor may be all that is necessary—or you might need to write them a detailed follow up letter. Don't underestimate the value of a well-researched letter to city hall, showing a need for a project and describing how it will improve the city while being cost-effective. You can also often make progress by testifying at city hall—extra points if you have business owners and other advocates lined up to give their testimony as well.

Politicians don't like to do anything without knowing that that they have citizen backup, and that the project will gain them more goodwill than criticism.

For that reason, among others, it is above all important to have, and prove, the support of the community for the project. To do this you need to actually make sure community members back you up. Listen very carefully to anyone who does not support or agree with you. If you can adjust your project or rhetoric to meet their needs, they might become allies instead of opponents. Even if this is not possible, you will likely have a good deal to learn from them.

Then, keep following up until the changes are made. Quite a bit of persistence is often necessary. If you run into roadblocks—either active opposition or simple inaction—don't give up. See the next section for more ways to demonstrate public support.

All of this is also true at the state and federal level. All you can do is learn everything you can, keep talking to people, keep your issue in the public eye, and persist until you make it. This may involve lawsuits, or trips to the capitol, or even launching major political campaigns—but those are all-consuming endeavors. Start small and you might be amazed by what you can accomplish.

Party Politics

Bicycle transportation is one of those rare issues that has appeal across all party lines. Liberals and conservatives can agree on the values of improving conditions for bicycling. Conservatives might be more inclined to point out the huge cost of our existing road system and the substantial economic savings, both individual and societal, as incentives to choose bicycling. Liberals might focus instead on the health, social, and environmental rewards of encouraging people to bike instead of drive. All points can potentially be agreed on across the board. If you're lucky, you live somewhere where bicycling has not become politically polarized. Otherwise, the best you can do is argue the case for bicycling on its merits and not play into the partisan arguments.

Bikes at Work

While many employers go out of their way to encourage employees to bike to work, many others are less inclined to provide material support such as secure parking out of the elements or places to shower and change after a long ride in. A few employers will even attempt to prevent their employees from riding.

If your employer doesn't encourage or actively discourages bicycling, it might be enough simply to ask for a change. On your own time, research bicycle parking costs and feasibility and present the plan to management. It might help to demonstrate the financial benefits that come from freeing up another car parking space, and presenting research about the benefits to employers in health care costs and productivity that stem from promoting active commutes.

If there are other bicycle commuters at your workplace, consider starting or joining a friendly

Business Case Study

In Portland, Oregon, the city's transportation department deployed a successful campaign to improve bike parking citywide. For years, a small bike parking fund has been available to install a bike staple that parks two bikes in the space between sidewalk and street for any business that requested it. The demand for bike parking had grown larger than these staples could accommodate, though, and some businesses were starting to demand more.

So the city set up a program to build "bike corrals," which replace one or two on-street car parking spots with between ten and twenty bike parking spaces. City transportation leaders signed up four prominent local businesses to test the program. When the plan was announced, there was considerable pushback from other business owners—losing car parking meant losing money, they declared.

The corrals went in and quickly filled with bikes. The initial businesses suddenly had more convenient parking spaces for paying customers, and other businesses almost immediately started demanding their own bike corrals. One restaurant owner started a petition. Now there are over 70 bike corrals throughout the city, with a long waiting list for more. Cities around the country are finding that installing bike corrals is one of the most affordable and politically feasible ways to encourage bicycling and give a boost to the local economy.

competition to log bike commute days or miles within the company or between different businesses. Building a culture of cycling will eventually make the case and create the demand for bigger changes in the workplace.

Businesses on Your Side

As you work to improve your city for bicycling, you'll find that local businesses large and small are among your strongest allies and your fiercest opponents.

When business owners, managers, and staff go out of their way to support cycling, even in small ways, let them know you appreciate it. Like politicians, business owners are much more likely to hear complaints than praise, and will often respond strongly to thanks—especially when those accolades are paired with an increase in visibility or customers.

Despite increasing evidence that cycling and walking customers tend to spend more than driving ones at downtown retail locations, many business owners are still skeptical of anything bicycle-related. Even the most anti-bike ones can often be won over, though. In these cases money may talk better than actual arguments. If a retail business is resisting bicycle facilities on their street, organize a ride with the purpose of visiting their business and spending money. Or ask everyone you know to go patronize the business, helmet in hand and ask the owner to support the bicycle improvements.

Sometimes a business owner might simply not be aware of cyclists' needs or that they are being friendly or unfriendly to them. For instance, if a delivery truck regularly parks in the bike lane outside a store, or the bike rack area is used to display merchandise, all you might need is a friendly letter to the owner letting them know that you support their business but need to have a safe and convenient way to park your bike there.

Bikes in the Media

When bicycle transportation makes it into the media, it isn't always in a positive light. We've all probably read at least one story in the local newspaper, or seen one on TV, covering a new bike lane, a bike event, or a crash in a way that doesn't seem to fairly portray cycling in general or a particular cyclist.

The good news is that as bicycling becomes more popular as a way to get around, media professionals are taking it up as well. But even if an individual reporter does ride a bike, their editor might not be bike-friendly—or a reporter in a hurry might just pull a story about a crash directly from the police reports, or a story about bicycle funding directly from a highway lobby press release.

It behooves bicycle riders to be alert and media-savvy in framing and responding to stories. When you're talking about bikes to the media, remember that you are telling a story more or less directly to people in your community. Imagine how you would talk about your cause to someone you know and respect, and tell the story that way.

Pitching the Media

One way to get realistic, positive stories about bicycle transportation in the news is to be proactive. Anyone can contact a reporter and suggest a story. Maybe you have an event, ride, or issue to publicize. If not, think about the most inspiring bicycle story you know. For instance, is your workplace or a local business especially friendly to bicycling? Or you can suggest yourself as a subject, focusing on how you work bicycle transportation into your life. This story will be most appealing if bicycling is unusual where you live, or if you do something outside the norm—for example, running a business by bike, biking with kids, commuting long distances, or carrying things that most people would assume requires a car.

Reporters will be more likely to cover your story if you make their job easier by giving them everything they need up front in a pitch. This includes a narrative for the story itself, which will preferably provide either an element of surprise, conflict, or overcoming obstacles. You'll also want to tell the reporter why their particular audience would be interested in the story and, if relevant, what section of their publication the story would be good for. Anything else you can provide that will help make the story quick and easy will make it that much more likely to happen—send quotations and photos to a blogger or newspaper writer; let a TV or radio editor know about strong visual or audio elements.

Then compile your pitch into an email of no more than three or four short paragraphs. Take some care with the wording; a hurried news outlet may simply copy and paste your words. Be sure to include your contact information as well as any necessary details about dates, times, and locations. If you aren't sure who to send your pitch to, call or email the news outlet with a quick question, like: "Who do I send a pitch about a family of six that gets around by bicycle?" If you are pitching multiple outlets, personalize each pitch and send them individually. When someone bites, get back to them quickly. Even if you don't hear a response, it's fine to send a follow-up email or reminder a week later.

Working with the media is all about developing relationships. When a reporter writes a story based on your pitch, thank them for their coverage. If you liked the way the story turned out, be sure to put them at the top of your list when you pitch future stories. Likewise, be sure to thank reporters and editors any time they provide positive coverage of bicycling.

Responding to Negative Press

When you see a story that seems unfairly negative or biased towards bicycling, there are several ways to respond.

If a basic fact is wrong, you can request a correction from the paper. If a major perspective in a story isn't represented, you can contact the reporter directly to fill in the gaps and let them know that there's more to the story than they might have initially uncovered. If you are friendly and provide good, concise information, the reporter might just call you up in advance the next time they are assigned a story about cycling.

You can also respond to a story, positive or negative, by writing a letter to the editor or leaving a comment on the online version of the story. When crafting these, it is best to be brief, informative, and levelheaded. Write a couple of drafts and let the final one sit for a while before posting or sending it. Make sure your facts are impeccable and your tone is confident and encouraging.

Remember that any time you speak or write publicly about bicycling, you will reach a large audience of people—including reporters and editors themselves—who may be hostile or uninformed about cycling now, but who have the potential to become sympathetic allies, and who are likely to start cycling themselves one day and forget that they ever thought of it as anything other than a joyful experience.

Conclusion

I was timid and tentative about cycling for many, many years. I didn't start to feel truly comfortable on a bike in traffic until I started spending time with other people who rode bikes every day. My new bike friends and I would ride through the city at night in search of empty streets and late night donuts, discuss turn signals on the Internet, argue over our favorite places to cross the interstate or get up the ridge in the northeast part of town, egg each other on to organize events or write letters to city hall.

Bicycling became a mark of pride for me, of identity and community. Being a cyclist inspired me to stop riding the bus or begging for rides from friends when I needed to get somewhere that had previously seemed too far away to bike. I began to apply for bike-related jobs, go on bicycle dates, write long op-eds about bicycle laws, infrastructure, and culture, and dedicate myself to learning about cycling and being a bicycle activist in every spare moment.

When I started to think of myself as a "bicyclist," I also started to notice that other friends who I'd known for years also rode bikes all the time. I invited one of these old friends on a group ride I was participating in, something silly involving costumes. She wasn't interested. "I don't want to be a cyclist," she said. "I just want to ride my bike to the grocery store."

For cycling advocates, this attitude is the ideal end goal: That getting around by bicycle becomes so normal that everyone can just get on a bike without thinking twice about it, changing their habits or identity, or reading a book like this one.

My dream is that within the next decade this book, along with the idea of identifying as a cyclist will be obsolete, a curiosity. I hope that someday soon, we will all start learning bicycle skills as young children, and that bicycling will become so normal that nobody has to think twice about it and that any adult still new to cycling will find themselves already surrounded by role models. I love the passion of my bicycle communities, but I envision the day when that energy and creativity can be directed elsewhere. That cultural shift is already happening, and by reading this book you are a part of it.

Now get out there and ride your bike!

Acknowledgments

This book owes all of its merit to the many, many people I've talked with and learned from about bicycling over the years, and particularly to the generous souls who shared their knowledge during the writing process of this book. All errors and omissions are purely my own.

The family bicycling chapter owes its existence to the wise words of friends and strangers. Special thanks to Katie Proctor for reviewing a very rough draft and making helpful suggestions, and to Kath Youell, Emily Finch, Kevin Turinsky, Nicole Donnelly, Chris Trahey, Travis Wittwer, Kristi Wood, Dan and Kirsten Kaufman, Doug Smart, Eric Moody, Madeleine Carlson, Stacy Bisker, and Sarah Noga for telling me their stories and lending their words to the text.

Caroline Paquette read two chapters in draft form and, once she stopped laughing, provided vital technical revisions. Sara Stout, Erik Sandblom, Lisa Finn, Miriam Rigby, Russ Willis, and Austin Horse lent their wisdom about some of the more vital myriad details.

Kate Berube and Meghan Sinnott typed several large chunks of the manuscript. Davey Oil did the dishes and imported much-needed good cheer during the final two weeks of writing. Taylor Hurley at Microcosm helped with edits for the second edition.

Joe Biel listened to every detail, believed in me every day, and is the reason this book exists in the first place.